# THE WOMEN'S POOL

# *The* WOMEN'S POOL

Edited by
Lynne Spender

SPINIFEX

First published by Spinifex Press, 2021

Reprinted 2022

Spinifex Press Pty Ltd
PO Box 5270, North Geelong, VIC 3215, Australia
PO Box 105, Mission Beach, QLD 4852, Australia
women@spinifexpress.com.au
www.spinifexpress.com.au

Copyright © on the collection Lynne Spender 2021
Copyright © on individual contributions remains with the authors
The moral right of the editors and authors has been asserted.

All rights reserved. Without limiting the rights under copyright
reserved above, no part of this publication may be reproduced,
stored in or introduced into a retrieval system, or transmitted,
in any form or by any means (electronic, mechanical, photocopying,
recording or otherwise) without prior written permission of both
the copyright owner and the above publisher of the book.

**Copying for educational purposes**
Information in this book may be reproduced in whole or part for
study or training purposes, subject to acknowledgement of the source
and providing no commercial usage or sale of material occurs.
Where copies of part or whole of the book are made under part VB
of the Copyright Act, the law requires that prescribed procedures
be followed. For information contact the Copyright Agency Limited.

Edited by Lynne Spender
In-house editing by Pauline Hopkins and Renate Klein
Cover design by Deb Snibson, MAPG
Typesetting by Helen Christie, Blue Wren Books
Typeset in Minion Pro
Printed by McPherson's Printing Group

A catalogue record for this
book is available from the
National Library of Australia

NATIONAL
LIBRARY
OF AUSTRALIA

ISBN: 9781925950458 (paperback)
ISBN: 9781925950465 (ebook)

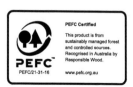

PEFC Certified

This product is from
sustainably managed forest
and controlled sources.
Recognised in Australia by
Responsible Wood.

PEFC

PEFC/21-31-16     www.pefc.org.au

*For women, everywhere*

# Contents

# Introduction:
# *The Women's Pool*

## Lynne Spender

ACKNOWLEDGING ELDERS — past, present and emerging — at the Coogee women's pool has particular resonance. It is rumoured that before colonisation the pool was a bathing and a birthing place for the Bidjigal and Gadigal women of the Eora Nation, who lived in and around the Coogee area. We have lost their stories, but acknowledge their enduring custodianship of the pool. Now, after a century of women managing the pool, this book pays tribute to the local women, many of them 'elders' too who have continued with both the guardianship of this special place and with the tradition of storytelling.

McIver's Ladies Baths is a sheltered rock pool, just south of Coogee beach. It is surrounded by native vegetation that is carefully nurtured by a bush care group. It's a sanctuary for women at all stages of pregnancy and except at the height of summer, it remains a peaceful, private, yet powerful place.

The pool has a rich history, reflecting women's status both as swimmers and citizens. Records indicate that colonists were bathing at the pool as early as the 1830s. Randwick Council oversaw the excavation of the pool and added the cement walls for its official opening in 1876 as a 'women only' space. The women only designation was not as a result of feminist activism. It was to provide access to swimming at a time when mixed bathing was frowned upon. In a memoir about the pool, Doris Hyde, daughter of the McIvers after whom the pool is named, gives at least one other reason. She refers to an article from the then *Eastern Herald*, which reported that it was the result of the Council receiving complaints that men were wilfully remaining in the vicinity of (mixed bathing) baths and were preventing the ladies and their attendants from bathing.

Olympians Fanny Durack and Mina Wylie swam and trained at the 30 metre women's pool at a time when regulations imposed by the NSW Amateur Ladies Swimming Association limited their entry to 'public' pools. The restrictions were based on concerns for modesty and fear of the exposure of women swimmers to what we would today perhaps call 'the male gaze'. Fanny and Mina attended the 1912 Olympic Games in Stockholm — the first games to admit women competitors — and won the gold and silver medals respectively for the 100 metres freestyle event. They became Australia's first swimming heroines.

Randwick Council handed the lease and management of the baths to Rose and Robert McIver, after whom the pool is named. In 1922, the Randwick and Coogee Ladies Amateur Swimming Club took over the lease and for many years ran free swimming lessons for children. Rose McIver, a staunch supporter of women's right to swim, remained actively involved. Now licensed to and managed by the Randwick & Coogee Ladies Swimming Association, the pool is still officially known as the McIver's Ladies Baths, but locals refer to it as 'the women's pool'. Its women-only status (accompanying children are also allowed) has been secured with a 1995 exemption from the NSW Anti-Discrimination Act. The story of the legal challenge by a Coogee man to his exclusion from the pool — and the fierce campaign run by women to preserve it as a women's space — is detailed in the book, as are tales of the vandalism and arson during the 1970s and 80s.

In 2020, strict COVID regulations disrupted the established rhythms of the pool and the income stream that sustains it. In 2021, another challenge arose: the legal and moral rights of transgender and transitioning people to access the pool. The challenge has also been faced by the Hampstead Ladies' Pond in London, and is indicative of the crucible for change that women-only spaces have become in a time of changing social mores relating to women's bodies. The trans women approached to include their stories in this collection declined to have their writing published in this book.

Most of the stories in the book are personal. They are impressions, experiences and recollections of time spent at the pool. Many are amusing, others are lyrical and reflective. All attest to the important role the pool has played in the lives of women, from diverse cultures and of different ages, who have prized it for over a hundred years as a sanctuary, a community and a place of natural beauty. In the summer of 2019, over 40,000 women from all walks of life and from many countries paid their small entry fee to experience the magic of the women's pool.

This book is an attempt to capture the spirit of the pool and of the women who have cared for it for generations.

*Lynne Spender*
*September 2021*

# *Cocooned*

## Therese Spruhan

IN SUMMER, when a good friend returns to Sydney from her home in London, we make an annual pilgrimage to McIver's Ladies Baths beyond the south end of Coogee beach. Each time we've visited I've discovered something new — the beauty around the shallow edges where the sandstone becomes a rainbow of pink, purple, orange and green; crabs crawling between crevices; limpets and zebra periwinkles that remind me of the aniseed boiled lollies my nana gave me when I was a kid. It's where I've felt as though I'm cocooned when I swim beneath the sandstone cliff that curves around the pool on one side, and where I've discovered an underwater rock that's weathered into the shape of a heart. It's also where one of the pool's custodians told me stories about the place — that it used to be a birthing area for Aboriginal women and that today it continues to hold the kind spirits of women past.[1]

---

1   *This extract was previously published in* The Guardian, *26 Jan 2020.*

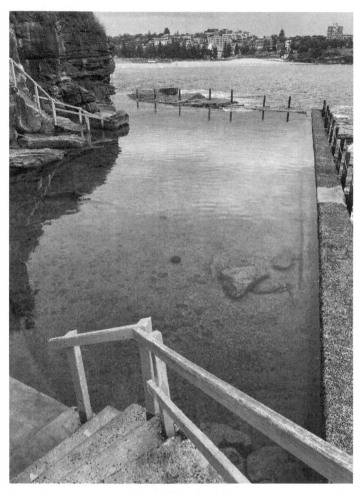

*The Women's Pool*
Photograph by Clarissa de Castro Lima

*Tess Durack, a writer, swimmer and confessed ocean lover, introduces her son to some of the pleasures — and mysteries — of the women's pool.*

# The Joys of the Women's Baths

## Tess Durack

"WHY AREN'T THERE ANY willies in here, Mum?"

Ah, yes. You can always depend on a pre-schooler to get straight to the point. At five years old, my son is young enough to still be allowed entry to the women's ocean pool and to get away with asking a question like that in a room full of half-undressed women. It's a good question. And a fair one. After all, this place is unique in that sense.

Nestled into the rocks, with the wide Pacific lapping at its walls, the pool glistens and ripples before us as we stroll down the path toward it.

On this warm, easy day, the array of bodies and ages and ethnicities at my beloved women's baths is a sight to behold: languid summer goddesses looking like mermaids just popped up from the ocean; elderly women who have been swimming here for decades; gaggles of hijab-wearing teenagers disrobing to their swimsuits and listening to

Taylor Swift on their phones; women recovering from injury or trauma, moving gently through the healing water and the sunshine.

Then there are the tired but happy new mothers floating calmly with their tiny babies as the local army of blue crabs makes its cautious march around the surrounding rocks. And women like me, relishing the chance to escape and let go of the demand to look and behave in certain ways. Just for an hour. Ahhh …

It's easy to guess at some of the reasons these girls and women might choose the baths, to imagine what they might be retreating from, protecting themselves against, taking comfort in, or nurturing strength for. My reason was pretty straightforward — I was weary of battling for lane space with large blokes at my local ocean pool. I was forever being overtaken with great thrashings of water as Kieran Perkins wannabes hurtled past me with windmilling arms, pounding legs and only centimetres to spare. I have had the back of my calves whacked by male swimmers surging up behind me before the last-minute manoeuvre, and ended up feeling like a small hatchback being tailgated, then overtaken, by a huge four-wheel-drive and left spluttering in its fumes.

I tried not to take it personally. They are just bigger and faster. But their supposedly 'innocent' lack of awareness was galling given the way I, like many women, never stop being aware and accommodating of other people, and alert to not 'getting in the way'.

So, one morning I ventured a few beaches further south to the women's baths and oh, what a gem of a place. There is not a tailgater in sight.

The roughly hewn ocean pool, with stairs leading down to two different entry points, is surrounded by an assortment of rock platforms and small grassed areas for general lolling about. There is also an outdoor shower among the nasturtiums, and a simple, clean, dressing room with a million-dollar view of the bay through its wide, open window.

The bottom of the pool is irregular and there are no marked lanes but those of us swimming laps stroke up and down smoothly enough in a natural synchronicity. Non-lap-swimming women bob graciously from our path. It's all so civilised! And so peaceful. There are many shared smiles of the "can you believe how gorgeous this is and how lucky we are?" type.

I am lucky in many ways, of course. One of which, to borrow from Virginia Woolf, is that I am in possession of a room of my own in which to write. The women's baths — well, they seem like something equally precious — a pool of our own in which to drift.

Don't get me wrong. I love a good beach session as much as the next person, and that frisson that accompanies the proximity of one's barely-clad body to other barely-clad bodies, against a backdrop of sand and surf, can be one of life's great pleasures. But being able to retreat from a state of hyper-awareness as to how I'm presenting my body, and how it's being perceived, is a huge relief. If a contented sigh could be manifested as a physical place, the women's baths would be it.

So back to my son's question. The simple answer is that there are no willies because there are no men allowed at the baths. My son's inevitable response to that is, of course, "But why?"

And as we walk back up the dappled path and out into the world, I take a deep breath. "Well," I begin ...[2]

---

2    *This article previously appeared in the* Sunday Life *magazine supplement of* The Sydney Morning Herald *and* The Sunday Age, *20 January 2019.*

*When grief about her mother's Alzheimer's was becoming overwhelming, Jane returned to the women's pool for solace. She writes eloquently of her encounter with the water and with women's bodies, including her own.*

# Morning Thalassa

## Jane Messer

YOU NEED THALASSA THERAPY, the woman said to me, knowing that I was ever so anxious and sad about too many things. These included my mother's months in hospital and her decline from Alzheimer's, made worse by all the stops and starts to any of us being able to visit her at the aged care home during COVID. I would weep in short sobs or just tears streaming, at any hour of the day. There was also the fraught health of one of my children. I'd wake in the middle of the night, with a ping of fright flowering in a burst in my sternum. At the university where I worked we were suffering endless rounds of workplace change, redundancies and the ominous morning emails from our Dean and Vice Chancellor. I was meeting each day with a feeling of dread.

To put it simply, there was a lot going on and it all involved uncertainty, worry and rarely, hope.

"In the early morning before the day has told you what it is going to be like, take yourself into the sea. Give yourself your *thalassa*," the kind woman told me. To give yourself *thalassa* therapy is simple. You walk into the sea, and immerse yourself, all of your body, from head to toe. The ancient Greek word *thalassa* simply means the sea. The Greek sea was a she, and Thalassa was her primeval spirit, and like the sea, her body was strong. She spawned both fish and storm gods. In some Greco-Roman mosaics she has the sharp horns of the crab claw. She is fish-tailed, her hair is black and thick. Dolphins, sea horses, octopus and fish swim with her.

It was to McIver's pool that I began to go for my morning *thalassa*. I wanted the calm waters of the women's pool, not the turbulent exuberance of the surf. I would arrive long after dawn on a weekday, but still early enough that the sun was slanting brightly along the pool's moving, shimmery surface. A friend came with me, a woman who has swum there countless times. She is sun-browned, creviced and wrinkled; lean and strong. She has walked up and down the steep steps to the sea pool many times. She'd slide into the water ahead of me then lap easily, for she's long been an ocean swimmer.

I didn't lap, not to begin with. I'd dip myself down, my toes feeling out the serrations of rock and shell, the silk of the weeds. I'd feel the sea water loosen and slide through my hair. I'd feel the change from air to water, from warm to cool, from business to being here, under the sea. Submerged, I'd open my eyes to look up through the water to the sky, my breath bubbling to the surface in pockets of light. The sea pool made my body my friend again. My body felt then that it had always been thus, for these few moments, lithe and buoyant, and almost joyful.

Over by the rocky undersea wall, live purple and black-spined sea anemones, barnacles, cockles, crabs, sometimes octopus, and sea urchins. Small fish dart about; Maori wrasse and Old Wives — fish that are plain grey and short-finned, or colourfully striped with fins that undulate. From the northern rock's overhang, water falls in precise droplets to the tiny rock pools below, each droplet arriving with a startlingly bright miniature splash. I would take a deep breath, dive, and swim across the rocky floor, then swivel with a twirl and lie on my back gazing, not breathing, letting the sea do its therapy.

Sometimes if it was early, there was just me and my friend, or another swimmer or two lapping, or a woman simply floating. There is a pool-net for sweeping up any blue bottles that have come in over the sea wall. One day my friend and I removed six. A woman in a floppy red hat was treading water slowly, gazing at the water, the mosses, at us doing this work, at nothing in particular. On a small square of concrete on the ocean side of the pool, a woman gracefully balanced on one leg in a slow tai chi dance. A dimpled Rubenesque woman stepped down the stairs holding her loose bare breasts in her hands, then let go when she reached the water. A young woman stepped out, water streaming as she shook her long hair. She climbed the stairs and sat above us, crossed-legged, facing the early morning sun to dry, like a cormorant.

The women on the rocky points remind me of basking seals, round and gleaming with oil or water, or of sea birds drying their wings before the next dive. I have seen so many bodies here: wrinkle-bummed, wobbly-bummed, long-breasted, with shell-white skin, and skin that is mottled from a lifetime of use. You can tell who the ocean swimmers are if they're a bit older because they have lean arses and strong shoulders and invariably wear Speedos. When I shower, peeling off my swimmers, rinsing my hair and skin in the cold water, then walking to one of the benches where my clothes lie in a tumble, I feel a little embarrassed that I have almost no pubic hair now, whereas my friend, who is much older than me, still has hers. Is she still, after all these years, naturally brown? I could dress in the privacy of one of the change rooms, but that would be missing the point. I seem to have become like my late godmother. I saw her sparse white hairs once when she'd accidentally left a button undone on her 'housedress'. I now remind myself of her, or of an old dog's grey snout.

On sunny weekends, groups of women in twos and threes will tread carefully across the rock platforms looking for an untaken space to sunbake. Out come the towels, the cool drinks and fruit, the sunblock and hats. One time I watched a black-haired woman reveal herself as a toned athlete in an apple-green G-string. Then she folded her hijab away into her beach bag and lay back.

The Baths welcome us to its shelves of stone and grass for drying off, to doze, to talk, to preen, to gaze into the aqua green, ivory and midnight blue pool, to the rocks and outcrops either side, and the Pacific Ocean beyond.

I wish I could bring my mother here. The minutes of joy and refreshment that I experience now in my morning swims, I wish my mother could have them too. Not that she likes cold water, or wind coming off the ocean. She has always been confident in her body, walking about unabashed from bathroom to bedroom, stopping on the way to say something to her cringing daughter. As a girl unwillingly becoming a young woman, I was horrified by the ever-so-slight sag of her stomach and gnarly brown nipples and the unapologetic lack of shame. The pool is the great leveller, welcoming the agile and the infirm, the exceptional and the ordinary. Much of the time I now gladly inhabit my body, that has borne children, braved surgeries, and most grievously, lost its beautiful, saucy oestrogen after menopause. The self-acceptance doesn't come easily. But I'm well aware every day that, all in all, my body has done me remarkably well so far.

At the pool there are no mirrors to see oneself in, other than the dappled water. There is much to *feel* there: your own salty skin and dripping hair, the ancient sandstone beneath your feet, the frisky embrace of the tidal sea water and ocean breeze. Swimming in the water I feel myself whole, from head to toe.

Rubbing my hair dry one time, feeling the sun-warmed towel on my cold scalp, I remembered a terrible moment a few months before, when my mother was still in the hospital. She had asked me, "Where is my head?"

"Your head? Your head is here," I said, touching her hair gently, expecting that once she felt the contact, she'd know it again.

"But, *where* is it?" she insisted. She has always been a conceptual person, interested in systems and relations. "It's at the top of your body, here where it always is, at the end of your neck," I said. I felt her confusion like a small, contained explosion within me. Another part of her mind had disassembled, fallen off like a loose rock might. Only when I crouched down in front of her, held her hands to anchor us both, and looked at her did she begin to reorient herself. "You're looking at me from your head, Mum," I said.

"That's right," she said, nodding. Everything was back in place again.

There are times in your life when you need help and nurture, and to feel safe. And so, I take my *thalassa* therapy, arriving before the day has told me what it is going to be like.

*Mother and daughter, Judy and Susan Banki, look forward to summer and to their delight in being together at the 'magical' women's pool. Susan tells of her dramatic attempt to discourage a male from entering the pool grounds.*

# Tides and Toms

## Susan Banki

LIKE THE ETERNAL RISE AND FALL of the tides, some things at the pool are bound to happen again and again. In the right months, patience while sitting on the rocks and gazing outward will yield the magical view of dolphins. On windy days, birds on the wing will push against that natural force, remaining stationary, right at level with our eyes. On hot summer days, picnics abound, while ants scurry to get morsels of baked bread with hummus, the discarded cherry stone, cheese rinds. A newbie uses her iPhone to take photographs, despite the written prohibition. On days with super swells, the pool is battered by crashing saltwater walls — it seems stingy to call these waves — while brave (foolhardy?) souls insist on dousing themselves, bobbing helplessly, as wiser women watch from the stairs, transfixed by the power of the sea, in a salty version of rubbernecking.

And, very frequently, a man will wander across the rocks in view of the pool. I am sure that some mean to spy, but most, I think, are simply unaware. Generally, a dramatic shooing gesture is sufficient to turn them away, but occasionally they aren't paying attention and make it all the way to the wooden beams and chains that delineate the pool itself.

On one such day I had just been for a run and joyfully entered the pool in nothing but my knickers: why ruin a perfectly good exercise bra with salt water when you can go topless, and feel the silk of the sea on your skin?

I entered the water, serene, and glided through the water with bent knees, keeping just my shoulders and head above water. Behind me, on the rocks and grass, dozens of women: some tattooed with cropped hair, some with children in tow, some who had been wearing a hijab until moments ago. All hoping to avoid the male gaze for at least a little while. And then I saw him: a perfectly harmless inattentive guy walking carefully on the rocks, his eyes trained on the slippery moss beneath him. Definitely not trying to perv, just having a meander on some rocks. I called to him, but he heard nothing. Waves too crashy. I signalled to him to do an about-face, but he was focused on his feet.

He finally got close enough and I shouted, "Ladies' pool!" He was puzzled. He just saw what looked to be a nice ocean pool. I gesticulated towards the fence, the cliffs, the few women in the pool at the moment, who, it so happened, were all in full bathing suits. I tried swirling my fingers around to show him: turn around and go.

But I could see on his face that he didn't get it. Why walk away from a lovely rectangle of ocean blue?

I could think of only one way to communicate to him that this wasn't just any ocean pool, but a place where women could feel safe, where they lounged in secret in open air. I straightened my legs, and enough of me rose from the water for him to see my decidedly unperky 50-year-old breasts.

That did it. He turned away with an embarrassed wave, and the ripple of discomfort at the pool smoothed out, like a tideless ocean, and the ladies' pool returned to perfect calm.

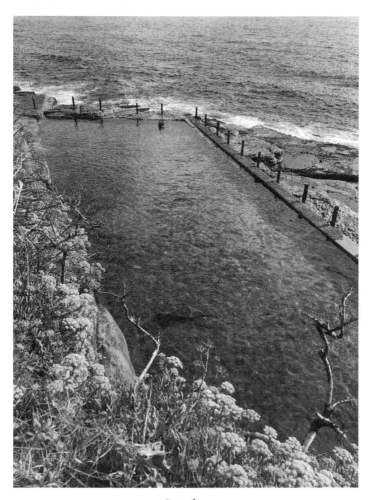

*Paradise*
Photograph by Jane Messer

*On one of her visits from New York to visit her daughter and family, Judy Banki, now in her nineties, describes her introduction to the paradise of the women's pool.*

# The Fabulous Ladies' Pool: Notes from a Non-Aussie

## Judy Banki

I DISCOVERED SUMMER IN AUSTRALIA about ten years ago, on a visit from New York to my daughter and son-in-law in Australia. I kept hearing talk about this magical women's pool, less than a ten-minute walk down the street from their apartment. "Wait till you see it," my daughter said. "You won't believe it." And so it was!

Descending the two flights of concrete stairs leading from the coastal walk to the entry platform of the McIver's Ladies Baths, I was struck by how magnificently beautiful the scene below was: a clear aquamarine rectangle, protected on two sides by high cliffs with stone staircases descending to the water, the other two sides consisting of rock walls fed by the ocean waves, which in stormy weather break against them, sending scallops of shining white foam into the pool.

21

The pool floor is the ocean floor: rocks and sand. Fish, tiny enough to fit between the spaces of the rock walls, dart back and forth. Black crabs scuttle across the stairs and landings. Occasionally, the alert goes out: "Bluebottles. Beware!" This stinging jellyfish whose tentacles import a non-lethal, but excruciating sting has found its way into the pool. Most of the women make room for an intrepid swimmer who comes down with a net and scoops up the intruder, to loud cheering and applause. It is rumoured that a blue-ringed octopus — lethally poisonous but shy — lives under some rocks near one of the two staircases leading to the pool.

Reserved for women and small children, the pool is an oasis of naked-to-the-bikini-line sunbathing for women of all ages and sizes. At the entry level, a change room, a free book exchange, a toilet and two cold-water showers. (In these, one may soap up and shampoo; an outdoor shower at the top of the staircases bears explicit no-nos: no soap, no shampoo, no conditioner: this shower drains directly into the ocean.)

Women are spread out on towels, blankets, mats, on the lawns, on flat-topped rocks along the water, some seeking shade, most seeking sun. A constant stream of women moves up and down the staircases: pre-teens, slim as reeds, in bikini bottoms; older women in regular bathing suits; devout Muslim women who swim with arms, legs and heads covered. Age and size do not determine body coverage. Some elderly and overweight folks, yours truly among them, swim and sun in bottoms; some perfectly-shaped bodies sport full body coverage. There is no dress code; there is no undress code (except bottoms must be covered, even if barely). Some come for a quick swim, others stay for the day, bringing family picnics. Many read, many text, some talk on the phone. Taking photos is prohibited, which makes a lot of sense; women who expose their upper bodies in the privacy of the enclave do not want to discover their boobs displayed on the internet. Occasionally, a male will penetrate the sanctity of the setting, approaching by foot, boat or jet ski; they usually get a finger from one of the women ranged along the side of the pool. Last week a young man in a bathing suit walked along the rocky shore, probably around the point from Coogee beach, to find himself on the edge of the pool. He grinned sheepishly as he was told to go back where he came from. These gals are cool; they do not panic easily.

I learn that the pool earned an exemption in 1995 from Australia's 1977 Anti-Discrimination Act. Some men are apparently incensed by that. Why should there be a women's pool when there are no pools restricted to only men? they complain. These macho types should learn a little history. Most pools in previous centuries *were* restricted to men. Women were allowed entry for just a couple of hours a day or perhaps one day a week. It was this outright and unjust discrimination that prompted Mrs McIver to ensure that the pool offered women and their young children the chance to swim safely and securely in a place that was said to be a traditional bathing place for Aboriginal women. Perhaps it is not a coincidence that the place turned out to be paradise.

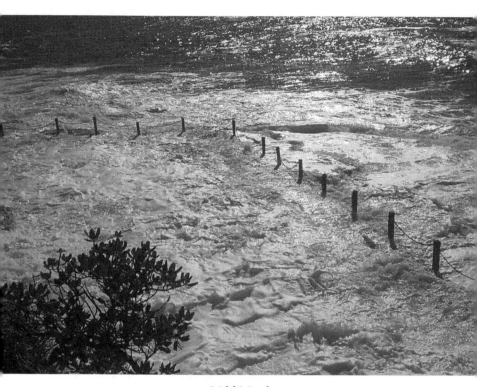

*Wild Weather*
Photograph by Wendy Freeman

*Mary Goslett is a Yuin Budawang woman who vividly connects the rhythms of Sydney's traditional Aboriginal seasons with those of the women's pool.*

# 'Women's Business'

## Mary Goslett

OUR BELOVED POOL is in D'harawal Country. A Land of six seasons, marked by the cyclical flowering of different plants, mating activities of mammals, and Law around traditional foods and ceremonial activities.[3] Since colonisation, the abundant sea life, the kangaroos, wallabies, quolls and echidnas have disappeared from our city coasts, but the women's pool still follows seasonal rhythms.

Non-Law people can easily dismiss First Nations culture and Law, because the uninitiated can know only a little of the layered complexity of a rich, nuanced culture that teaches belonging, respect, meaning and reciprocity.

Thus, Women's Business is often overlooked. In traditional Aboriginal society, daily routine sees women

---

3    D'harawal Calendar, Indigenous Weather Knowledge, *Commonwealth of Australia 2016, Bureau of Meteorology* <*http://www.bom.gov.au/iwk/ calendars/dharawal.shtml*>.

working and socialising with other women — and men with men — all coming together at the end of the day. This custom values difference and also shared experience, allowing space for integration as well as respect. As Hannah Bell explains, this division enables each to value the wisdom and power of the other, creates coherence between them and is fundamental to cultural harmony.[4]

Our pool is also a place of 'women's business', the interaction of women creating a melody of community and acceptance. Sometimes the low whistle and chortle of magpies can be heard, building to a mix of kookaburras and cockatoos. The ambient sounds both follow and presage the six annual seasons.

As I write, it's *Parra'dowee*. Warm and wet, from November to December, the time when summer heat starts to build and weather is largely stable. The great Eel Spirit calls his children to him. Eels, ready to mate, swim towards the ocean, down cool, dark rivers and creeks, shaking off the torpor of winter. *Kai'arrewan* (weeping Myall wattle) blooms, announcing populations of fish in the bay.

At the pool it's a time of startlingly-white skin (or suspiciously evenly-brown) that quickly turns scarlet. Bleary-eyed uni students straggle in like the precursors of migrating birds. Most squeal as they brave the water, shocked by the 17–18 degree chill. Beautiful sea slugs start to appear; sea lettuce wave underwater; the occasional rock cod is washed in and perhaps a small, bearded wobbegong.

---

4    Men's Business, Women's Business: The Spiritual Role of Gender in the World's Oldest Culture, *Hannah Rachel Bell, Inner Traditions/Bear & Co, 1998.*

Westerly winds flatten the ocean and swimmers can investigate rocks and crevices that are usually thumped by waves and are too dangerous to explore. Intrusive jet skis sometimes blast by, disturbing the peace. On very hot days the cultural diversity of the visiting women increases, and different tongues create polyphonic harmony.

The season of *Burran* is next: January to March. It's hot and dry and the Sydney basin swelters. The water feels like liquid silk, and early morning swims are magical — until the crowds build. *Weetjellan* (hickory wattle) blooms and male kangaroos become aggressive and territorial, as do some of the males of the human species who challenge their exclusion from the pool, or leer from the path above. Nor'easters bring shoals of bluebottles, Portuguese man-o-wars that are rapidly scooped out but eventually arrive in overwhelming numbers. On sweltering hot days, only the bravest do a very quick dip.

As the heat of the day builds, the surrounding sandstone rock shelf resembles a seal colony, with every inch of open space fiercely coveted. Women arrive and arrive, now necessitating a head count and pool closure when numbers become unsafe. Some days there is standing room only in the pool. People liberally slather or spray themselves with sunscreen and then dive in and wash it off. By afternoon, there can be a deep layer of floating scum.

In the following season of *Marrai'gang*, from April to June, our Country becomes wet and cool. On the shores, the cry of the *Marrai'gang* (quoll) seeking a mate could once have been heard. As lilly pillies ripen and daylight saving ends, locals breathe a sigh of relief and again we can do our laps easily. Water is still warmish and the chill of the air freshens rather than oppresses.

Beautifully clear, sunny Sydney days line up like jewels, and both sea and sky are an exquisite rich blue. Snorkelling is delicious; visibility feels endless, and blue gropers and zebra fish proliferate in the deeper water off the rocks. The briny smell thickens and deepens. When the fruits of the lilly pilly start to fall, traditional owners mend old cloaks or make new ones. At the pool it's too cold to sit in your wet cozzies after a swim.

The time of *Burrugin*, cold and frosty, is June to July. The water chills to the bone. We talk of 'night water' when the pool has settled at night and is not yet warmed by the sun. Even serious swimmers don swimming caps and socks.

*Burrugin* is when we reassure ourselves that our resident octopus is alive and well. A common Sydney octopus, he can be seen below, cleverly camouflaged and incredibly alert. Whales swim north to warmer waters, and a pool visit feels complete when we witness a breach or even just a spout. Once, male echidnas, *Burrugin,* formed lines in the foreshore bush, eagerly following the females in their attempts to mate. The *Burringoa* (ironbark) starts to flower, announcing the need to gather different nectars for ceremonies in the season to come.

*Wiritjiritbin* time is cold and windy, from July to August. Lyrebird builds his dancing mound and his mating calls ring out in the bush. The *Marrai'uo* (wattle) starts to blossom, signalling the running of the fish in the rivers. Swimming at the pool becomes a mystical experience in the cold and in the rain, every single raindrop visible as it hits the water.

Some days it feels like it will never be warm again. Even the most hardened locals huddle in the open doors of the change cubicles to escape the wind and rain.

During *Wiritjiritbin*, the cold water outdoor shower feels warm. Hypothermic clumsiness makes it difficult to get dressed. In the storms, the waves crash on the rocks at the back of the pool. Flotsam and jetsam wash turbulently in and out. The oceanscape is spectacular, the wildness filling your soul. Sometimes you can experience the joy of being a lone swimmer.

At the end of *Wiritjiritbin*, the *Boo'kerrikin* (black wattle) flowers to announce the changing season, and gentle spring rains arrive. They herald *Ngoonungi*, September to October when it's cool, becoming warm. Flying foxes gather across D'harawal land and dance through the sky just after sunset; day lengthens, and daylight saving brings longer opening hours at the pool. The 'seals' return in twos and threes to spread their multi-coloured towels across the rocks.

In pockets of uncleared bushland, bright red *Miwa Gawaian* (waratah) flowers appear, signifying the heat to come. At the pool, those in the know pick the flowers of the introduced nasturtium and add them to their salads. Superb blue fairy wrens dance and flirt; the haunting and annoying calls of the common koels are heard late at night. It is a wonderful season of luxuriating in the warmth of the sun knowing that the chill of the water means little competition for a solo swim. Whale spotting is even more exciting, as calves accompany adults on their trek south. If we are lucky, we see both whales and dolphins.

Then we are back to *Parra'dowee*. The ancient seasonal cycles find their own rhythm at our pool, at our place of 'women's business.' In the vastness of this continent, it is a tiny space of companionship if wanted, or solitude if needed. Where women can heal and rest and play and feel safe. A sacred space of rejuvenation and sisterhood, simply respecting the feminine.

*A Vietnamese-born pool regular tells of the role water has played in her life and the role of the women's pool in her valiant attempts at learning to swim. She wishes to thank Wendy A for providing some advice on sentence structure. And to thank Carol C for teaching her to swim.*

# Lai Learns to Swim

## Lai Nguyen

MY BIRTHPLACE IS A SMALL VILLAGE in South Việt Nam, surrounded by a network of tributaries of the Mekong River. Prior to 1975, the Vietnamese government had been involved with war matters, and had not developed roads and infrastructure, so the only routes into and out of the village were by boat.

From early days, water was part of my life. As children, my sisters and I would take the family's washing to the river, and we would step in near the riverbank to wash the clothes. Our mum was very strict, and implored us not to try swimming. An older sister had nearly drowned when she went in too deep, and our mum instilled in us a great fear of the water. Mum was of Chinese ancestry and very traditional. She did not think girls needed to learn much academically, but I sailed through school and came top of the class in maths and other subjects. I begged and begged her to let me study further, and due to my determination and the fact that I was the youngest and there were still some other sisters at home, she eventually relented.

I didn't know when I left home in 1970, aged 16, that the water that led me to Saigon to continue my studies would be both the opportunity and the symbol for my transformation. As the local boat left the village, with me on it, and we travelled downstream with familiar dense jungle on either side, I was overwhelmed with excitement about how my life was about to change. As the river got wider, and the landscape more open, I wondered what urban living would bring. I ended up studying chemical engineering at university. I also met the man who would ultimately become my husband.

On 30 April 1975, the Vietnam War ended, but it did not bring the kind of peace that we had dreamt of. My country was in a total economic downturn, controlled by foolish communists vowing to take revenge on us. We did not want to die there, so began making plans to escape. Again, water played a role in my transformation. However, instead of peacefully chugging down the alluvial Mekong with fellow villagers and bags of books, this time we were crammed into a fishing boat, crouched under canvas covers, where we were hidden, but terrified that we would be caught — surely a fate worse than death. It was 1985 and after several aborted attempts to leave, I found myself packed in very tightly with my teenage niece and around 30 other escapees whom we did not know. All had paid large sums for this dicey exit card. We had only the clothes we were wearing.

As we lurched and pitched out of the estuary into the open sea, many succumbed to sea-sickness. We still had several days ahead of us, but once we had made it out of the territorial waters, we were allowed to crawl out from under the tarpaulins and witness the South China Sea for the first time. I was happy to feel the fresh salty air and see the sky, but also petrified, as the 12-metre boat was old and rickety, with only a small antiquated engine, and I doubted whether it would survive the voyage. Furthermore, there were pirates to contend with, and other unspeakable terrors waiting for the 'boat people', as Vietnamese refugees like us were known. One horror succeeded another as days and nights went past — sea-sickness, sunburn and fear of drowning were the least of them. Just as we were feeling utterly helpless, out there with nothing to see but ocean and waves, some birds appeared, and this was the first sign of hope. It took us another whole day to see land. We eventually made it to a Malaysian island, Pulau Bidong, and a refugee camp. We were so, so grateful to survive. Many others didn't.

The terror of the sea followed me for many years, and the difficulties of settling into Australia kept me busy. I got married (my husband had made it to Sydney ahead of me, via a different route). I raised two boys in Fairfield, made money by sewing at night when the children were young, and then got a job as a laboratory assistant at the University of NSW. I also became sick with cancer, struggled through treatment, somehow survived this too, and went back to work. In 2009, my family moved to Coogee. I had heard there were health benefits from living by the ocean.

My boss at work, in the laboratory, was a woman a little older than me. She had suggested that post-cancer therapy should include plenty of exercise and swimming in salt water. Her husband had also been sick, and had found these activities beneficial. I explained that I couldn't swim, but one hot morning in summer, close to Christmas, she took me to her favourite local swimming spot: McIver's Ladies Baths. I remembered my mother saying that daughters should never show their bodies in public, even under swimsuits, so I felt nervous. Too nervous even to notice quite how beautiful the rock pool was.

This first time, I wore shorts and a t-shirt. I went down the steps into the shallow area of the pool. My boss had brought along her grandson's polystyrene swimming float, but all I could do was stand in the water and marvel at the sensation of dipping my whole body in cold sea water. I was instantly addicted. Transformed. Desperate to learn to swim!

I bought a swimsuit, hoping my mum would not fidget in her grave. (After all, it was only other women at this pool, not men.) I also purchased a child's inflatable swimming ring. I started going to the pool and just standing in the shallow water, wearing the buoyancy aid. I jumped up and down a bit, but was terrified that if I put my face in the water, I would not be able to breathe, and would probably drown. I decided to enrol in a rather expensive 'Learn to Swim' course at the university aqua-centre. The classes involved a lot of holding the side and kicking practice, but, even by the end of the course, I still felt I had a long way to go before I'd be able to swim.

In the meantime, I kept visiting the ladies' pool whenever I could, and the more I went, the more I loved its gorgeous water that made me wish to stay in it forever; its beautiful view that helped me relax; and its friendly environment, created by a group of kindly volunteer ladies who managed and looked after the pool. I felt accepted and cared for.

One of these women told me that there were free swimming lessons at the pool on Saturday mornings, and I made an appointment to meet Carol, the instructor. Later, I discovered that she was also the president of the ladies' swimming club. These lessons were one-on-one, totally individualised, and so much more useful than the ones at the aqua-centre.

Putting my face in the water was still daunting, but I had the bright idea of acquiring a snorkel. I pronounced it *snoggle*, which made the other ladies laugh, but in a kind way. Some tried to help me with my still poor pronunciation, and I realised that this pool was not just used for swimming, but was also a place in which to enjoy the helpfulness and good humour of women.

For my next swimming lesson, I put on my swimsuit, snorkel, mask and inflatable ring, and — with Carol's gentle encouragement — I bravely immersed my face and kicked my legs. And kicked and kicked. But, annoyingly, I didn't move forward. Worse, when I was tired from kicking and wanted to stand up, I was alarmed to find that the inflatable ring kept my legs afloat against my will, and I was unable to put my feet back on the floor of the pool. (How was it that I couldn't control my body, and how could swimming be so difficult? Everyone else was doing it! Why not Lai?) Carol was patient and set me on course, and said how determined she thought I was. That motivated me to continue.

By the third lesson, I was *almost* 'swimming', and was undoubtedly advancing through the water — not just thrashing my arms and legs around on the spot, or going in circles. Carol told me to relax, and to imagine the rhythm of music as I moved my arms overarm. One, two ... One, two ...

Suddenly, I found I was *actually* swimming. What a wonderful feeling! The water was holding me up and I was enjoying it: the water was my friend, not my enemy. I was truly transformed.

AT AGE 56, LAI COULD SWIM!!!!

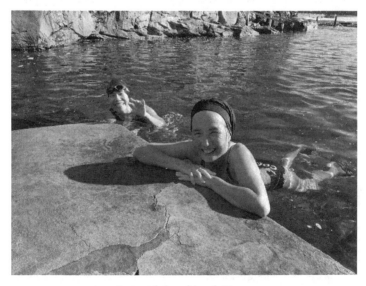

*Lai with her friend, Trang*
Photograph by Wendy Assinder

*COVID-confined to Scotland where she is caring for her mother, Grace Barnes explores the many connections between women and swimming.*

# Shifting Sands

## Grace Barnes

WHEN I ARRIVED IN SYDNEY FROM SCOTLAND in the late 1980s, I was captivated by the patches of glittering aquamarine which seemed to populate every park, every suburb. I became like the swimmer in John Cheever's iconic story, as I explored this shining city through the pools of North Sydney, Drummoyne, Surry Hills and the Domain. I delighted in seeing my arm pull through a shaft of sunlit water, and regularly switched to backstroke to marvel at the new sensation of watching flying birds instead of staring at an uninspiring roof. I discovered the city beaches and bodysurfed and dived through shoals of silver fish but, being wary of both sharks and surfers, I never attempted to swim from one side of Bondi to the other. Astonishing as it seems to me now, I had no awareness of the jade treasures of ocean pools which linked into an exquisite bracelet along the city's eastern coastline, and it took an announcement from my ferociously feminist housemate, Jackie, to bring them to my attention. "We're going to the women's pool," she said, in a manner that made it clear there was to be no argument. If someone had asked me to imagine the perfect place to swim, I could not have come up with an image as magical and as lovely as McIver's Baths in Coogee. How had this been here all the time and I had not known about it? More to the point, how could I go back to a chlorinated 50-metre tank after experiencing the unadulterated bliss of a sea pool? As if the natural beauty of this secret place wasn't enough, the fact that it was restricted to women enhanced the sensation of being in a special place. I was told that centuries ago, Aboriginal women considered the rock pool a sacred space and came here to bathe and conduct women's business, and as I lay on the grass that sunny afternoon, I too recognised the attraction of a women-only space. A place where women can just be, for once spared the obligation to either conform or perform.

I was embarrassingly apolitical in those days, but I listened, intrigued, as Jackie spelled out the importance and the wider significance of female only space. How men assume it is their right to occupy space in a way that women never do. How certain places — pubs, sports grounds, the beach — were assumed by men to be their domain and women thus became uninvited, and unwanted infiltrators. There, 30 years ago, amidst the gentle music of women's voices and lapping water, the first stirrings of feminist fury kicked like a foetus growing inside. Perhaps the residue of the secret ceremonies conducted here by the Aboriginal women had permeated the rocks and infused the water in the pool in order to empower each and every woman who immersed herself in its depths.

I carelessly lost touch with Jackie in those pre-internet days, but one winter morning, many years after my Coogee initiation, she found me in the shallow end of the heated Leichhardt pool, still meticulously timing my 200 metre sets. As I sit here now, remembering the hundreds of laps we subsequently swam together, it occurs to me that my swimming companions have always been women. Right back to my mother who taught me to swim in a pool in Spain when I was around five or six. When I became a member of the county swimming squad in Scotland, I was aware that my competition placings meant as much to Mum as they did to me, and she diligently drove me to training sessions through dark Scottish mornings. She even became a competition timekeeper, decked out in regulation whites and huddling in a group comparing the minute hands on stopwatches. It wasn't a coincidence that when I stopped competing in my late teens, Mum hired a coach to correct her technique and became an obsessive swimmer, often doing laps twice a day. I know now she was trying to freestyle herself out of a black depression, an unshakeable sense that life had passed her by, and it was all too late.

My first swimming friend was Susan, a backstroker on the county team who did not possess the driving need to win that I did. I liked Susan. I liked her honesty and her ability to listen. But it mattered desperately to me that I beat her at her own stroke, and if she had ever taken my freestyle title from me, the friendship would not have survived. When I was researching a PhD on the life of early swimming champion

Mina Wylie (from Wylie's Baths, a stone's throw from the women's pool) I became intrigued by the relationship between Mina and her contemporary, the more widely remembered Fanny Durack. After blitzing the inaugural 100 metres freestyle for women at the 1912 Stockholm Olympics, Fanny winning gold and Mina silver, the two swimmers became the first female sporting celebrities in Australia and were invariably referred to in the press as best friends. I was never convinced. My experience with Susan proved to me that a rival is a rival, and friendship counts for little when the county or state championship is at stake. It is generally men — boring husbands and controlling boyfriends — who are the greatest threat to female friendship, but I'll put money on it that Mina and Fanny's later estrangement was connected to their swimming careers.

Funnily enough, I learned to swim properly in a segregated space — a small pool, now long gone, reserved exclusively for women and girls in an imposing Victorian building on Edinburgh's seafront. I discovered however, that in Australia in the last decade of the 1800s, when sea bathing was undergoing an explosion in popularity, the mingling of the sexes in the newly built swimming enclosures was out of the question.

Victorian morality decreed that the kind of woman willing to flaunt her half-naked body in front of strangers belonged either on the stage or in a brothel. Public pools were therefore exclusively for men or for women, or had allocated hours for each sex, with men, naturally, given priority. Women who rode the tram to Coogee in the early 1900s stepped from the carriage and turned south towards the women's pool, while men made for Giles Baths on the northern cliffs. This state of affairs continued until 1912, when the inclusion of Mina Wylie and Fanny Durack in the Olympic swimming team inadvertently brought about the advent of mixed bathing in public pools in NSW.[5]

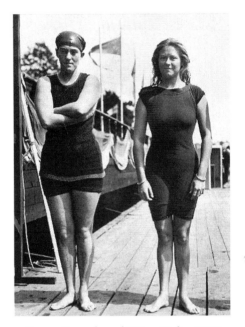

*Fanny Durack and Mina Wylie, 1912*
Photograph courtesy of Alamy

Rose and Robert McIver, however, continued to operate Coogee women's pool as a single sex facility, and when the lease was taken over by the Randwick and Coogee Ladies Swimming Club in 1922, there was no reason to change

---

5   *Wylie's Baths, next door to the women's pool, was the first public pool in Australia to offer mixed bathing.*

the status quo. A first attempt in 1946 to widen admission to both sexes was quashed by the Mother Superior of the nearby Brigidine Convent, who argued that the nuns and the students needed privacy to swim. She was supported in this by none other than Mina Wylie, although whether this was due to feminist convictions or a fear of a loss of income to the family business next door is anyone's guess.

I swam at Wylie's Baths with Lou, a talented but troubled filmmaker who disappeared into a fog of alcohol and unfulfilled potential years ago. I counted laps with my sister under the Aqua Profundo sign at Fitzroy Baths. I went on a swimming holiday to the Mediterranean and befriended the prickly American, Rosemary. One glorious afternoon off the island of Gozo, the rhythm of our strokes synchronised perfectly and we grinned in recognition every time our eyes met as we turned our heads to take a breath.

Women behave differently when men are not around, and the segregation of pools in the early days of swimming actually contributed to the popularity of the sport amongst women. In spaces such as McIver's Baths, women could not only free themselves from the physical restrictions of the tightly laced corset and the frills and cuffs and buttons, they could disregard the Victorian ideals of ladylike behaviour and engage in boisterous physical activity away from disapproving male eyes. In doing so, women came to discover that their bodies were not as weak, and their constitutions not as frail, as they had been led to believe. I love looking at photographs of early women swimmers in Sydney and trying to comprehend the sense of exhilaration that this physical and emotional freedom would have induced. I wonder if male authorities suspected that the sensuality of being fully immersed in the ocean would be a more intense experience for women, and keeping them apart was bound up in an innate fear of women's sexuality.

Annette Kellerman, the 1920s Hollywood aquatic star, declared swimming an activity more suited to women than men. Although her observation was influenced by the ideal of unthreatening femininity embodied by the graceful ballerina and the elegant figure skater, she was clearly aware that men and women swim differently. Men do battle with the water, crashing down lanes with aggressive splashing. Women, as ever, negotiate. Then make friends and play with the water, as equals. Swimming can be meditative in a way that other exercise is not, and perhaps women need bursts of mental solitude in a more visceral way than men do. Perhaps that is why they continue to come to the women's pool, and relish the calm, the gentleness of a space in tune with their need for reflection. For peace. Part of the joy of swimming, for me, is the silence. The space between the breaths filled with nothing but the splash of my hand hitting the water, and my own thoughts. Sometimes, I swear I can hear the sand shifting beneath me.

⤸

Back in my hometown in Scotland, I run into Susan at the gym and we are enthusiastic about getting together for a glass of wine. But we never do it. Jackie and I reconnected and watched the swimming competition at the 2018 Brisbane Commonwealth Games together (I have the selfie with Ian Thorpe to prove it). Rosemary and I are emailing about swimming the Bosphorus Strait. My mother now lives in the twilight zone of dementia. I take her to the local pool to watch the swimmers and she sits in her wheelchair gazing at the changing patterns of fluorescent light dancing on the water.

"This is lovely," she says, with no recollection at all of the hours she spent in there.

"Lovely."

*Josi Crow is in a rage about the pool signage. She won't be fined and towed away.*

# Signs of the Times

## Josi Crow

WHAT IS IT WITH THE SIGNS, LADIES? What's been happening while I've been gone?

When I hit the pool after too long away, what I see first are a dozen laminated, metal and sticker signs about what to do, and what not to do. How far apart to stand. The COVID safe policy. Nudity — none allowed, naturally. What knickers to wear. (Just kidding.) They begin as a cluster on either side of the gateway, then spread themselves out down the path to the payment booth. Someone tells me there are more than 40 signs at the pool. Signs about checking in, payment, hand cleaning, more about nudity, more about COVID.

I'm just here to swim, gals. Signs repeat the same information already on a sign just a metre away. Does Randwick Council think women are stupid? That we don't read? Do we need to be told, two, three, four times? I mutter something surly and a sweet-faced patron, unafraid to talk to me, says it's not Randwick Council that put up the signs.

"Who then?" I ask. "Who?"

"The women's pool executive," she whispers.

"Who are they?" I ask.

She shrugs, gamely.

I stand there five seconds more, getting myself worked up and septic. There's hardly anyone here. I read a sign about how many women are allowed in at one time: how many in the water, how many on the grass. I'm going to be allowed 30 minutes somewhere.

I'm bailing, I'm going to Wylie's instead. It's a pool a few hundred metres along the Coogee headland path. At Wylie's I find there are fewer signs, but more people — both women and men — which makes that pool, you'd think, far more complex to manage. Fewer signs. Weird.

A few days later I'm down at McIver's again. I'm itching over the signs, but I'm promising myself I'm not going to scratch. It's a red-pepper hot day in Sydney. I ignore the signs on my way in, ignore them on the path down towards the steps. I ignore the signs as I pass the change room and the shower. I focus on the colour of the little 'paddle' I've been given that helps the staff know how many women have come in.

I am woman. I am one. My 'paddle' is yellow. I promise I will hand it back when I leave.

I splash around in the cool pool for a bit. Sweet water! Then I notice the really tall metal signs. One on the south rock platform, one on the north platform, both facing towards me. These signs have been *cemented* into the ancient Gondwanaland sandstone rock.

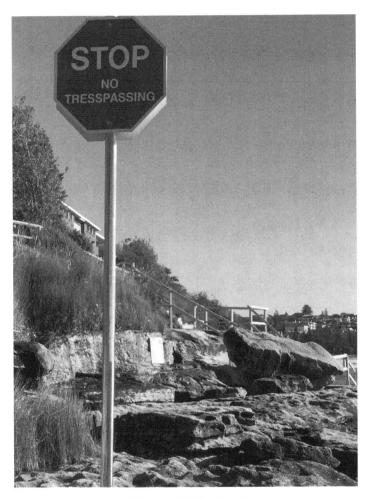

*What's with the signs?*
Photograph by Wendy Freeman

## STOP
### NO TRESSPASSING

Misspelt signage. They're red and white metal. RTA style. Very official, like No Parking. No Standing. Clearway. You will be fined and towed away.

No Trespassing? This is not the work of #landrightsnow. What the f—? Weird.

(*Girls*, pay attention. *Girls,* don't be naughty. *Girls,* you're not listening!)

At the #march4justice[6] this week, loads of marchers carry signs. The signs are made of cardboard, paper, packing tape, Texta and poster paints. Women have made these signs with their bare hands. These signs tell powerful, important messages:

"*I march for my daughters and yours too.*"
"*I wanna walk through the park in the dark.*"
"*Sick of rape culture? #MeToo*"
"*Our bodies Our Power No means No.*"

I don't carry a sign at the march. I'm a digital native. Can't do craft. Not the sign-making type. But I'm appreciating these signs. Especially:

"*I am rage.*"

After the march, I go home and rewrite my previously tame pool piece, to this one.

---

6    *The national #marchforjustice took place on 15th March 2021.*

*Yusra Metwally tells of her determination to rekindle her love of swimming and of her sheer delight at discovering the safe and nurturing space of the women's pool.*

# My Swimming Journey

## Yusra Metwally

ON THE FIRST DAY of autumn, complying with McIver's Baths new COVID-safe policies, I stand in line, 1.5 metres away from a mother with her chubby baby in polka-dot swimmers. I am excited about releasing the stresses of the day in the salty rock pool but my mum-guilt voice regrets not bringing my toddler to this special place. I tell myself that this is my '*mum-me*' time and I can't give from an empty cup. I made sure I brought my coins with me. However, COVID-19 has revolutionised the operation of the baths. A new cashless payment system means throwing a coin through the entry doors is now a thing of the past. The days of searching every nook and cranny of my car for coins are well and truly over.

McIver's is a place where I track my swimming journey from once being a non-swimmer, lazing around on the rocks and embracing rare suntanning opportunities. I'd have a dip in the water but never a serious swim. As I began to take ocean swimming more seriously, I swam laps in this outdoor, saltwater pool, allowing my body to be hugged by the coolness of the water. I developed a new-found appreciation for McIver's with its harmonious co-existence of swimmers and non-swimmers, without white marked lanes or lifeguards.

I've grown up with a love of the ocean and swimming. However, like many other Muslim women, my relationship with swimming became complex when, as a teenager, I started wearing the hijab as an expression of my faith. I was self-conscious about swimming in a public pool, especially in a top-to-toe black burkini. Sadly, it meant that I never attended a school swimming carnival. Back then, the burkinis on the market didn't speak to my style as a teenager and I tried to avoid wearing them. This was before modesty fashion became a multi-million dollar industry and long before model Halima Aden made history wearing a burkini on the front cover of *Sports Illustrated*.

When I was nine years old, my parents decided to move back to Egypt, after migrating to Australia in the1980s. I was so excited to have a pool inside my new school. On a hot Egyptian summer's day, I wore shorts and a 'rashie' that still had the scent of chlorine from Greenacre pool where I learned to swim. I put on my cobalt blue rash shirt with floral printed sleeves and my black swimming shorts. To my utter dismay, the Egyptian swim teacher took a look at me and told me that I couldn't swim in *those clothes*. She pointed to what I should be wearing, as modelled by my classmates who all wore one-piece swimsuits. That was the only form of swimsuit allowed, apparently for reasons of hygiene.

I was dumbfounded, disappointed and distraught. Yet I was too afraid to speak up and didn't have the confidence to argue against the stern teacher, nor did I have a strong enough grasp of Arabic to string my thoughts into a sentence. I sat on a wooden bench as I watched my classmates enjoy their swim. Splashes of water near my foot were as close to the water as I was going to get. After the hour-long drive home on a hot bus, I cried to my mother who immediately arranged to meet with the school principal to advocate against this swimming injustice. She challenged the 'hygiene' argument by telling the principal that my swimwear was recommended for children in the western democratic country, Australia, because it provided adequate UV protection. In hindsight, this experience sowed the seeds for my advocacy for women and swimming.

We returned to Australia in 2000, just before the Sydney Olympics when Ian Thorpe donned his full-body performance swimsuit, which, ironically, resembles a burkini. But for Muslim women, swimming in the burkini swimsuit unintentionally becomes a political act. Despite the fact that an Australian, Aheda Zanetti, invented the burkini to make swimming accessible for Muslim women, my burkini invites questions and sometimes confusion, whether in Granville in the heart of Western Sydney, or at the iconic North Sydney Olympic pool. For years, I aimed to get to the local Granville pools for a 5 a.m. swim squad, run by a triathlon club. When I did — and walked around the pool looking for the group while it was still dark — I was asked by a 70-year-old man in budgie smugglers: *"What are you wearing?"*

The feeling of being policed at pools continued into my adolescent years. I recall being at the Sydney Olympic Aquatic Centre on a hot day. A lifeguard approached to tell me that I wasn't supposed to be swimming in non-lycra material and I was asked to get out of the water.

Despite the barriers, I persevered with swimming because I craved the feeling of being at one with the water by swimming smoothly and harmoniously, rather than gasping for air whenever I attempted to swim freestyle. I loved the feeling of being hugged by the coolness of the saltwater and valued the sense of freedom, calm and serenity that swimming brings. I felt an overwhelming desire to continue swimming and add ocean swimming to my bucket list, despite not being able to freestyle properly. I was inspired by the story of an Olympic swimmer who shared my first name, Yusra Mardini. As a teenager escaping Syria, she spent hours in the Aegean Sea, swimming to assist a broken-down refugee boat to safety.

I thought I could simply sign up to an ocean swim training program, but realised that I needed to improve my swim skills. I took advantage of the allocated two hours per week of 'WimSwim' lessons held at Roselands Leisure and Aquatic Centre, where I could swim in a one-piece bathing suit in a women-only session. I knew I needed to have the confidence to swim outside of these sessions so swimming in the outdoor 50-metre pool was the next hurdle. It was intimidating to swim in a pool with marked lanes while also being conscious of my slow speed, my shoddy technique and lastly, standing out in my burkini. But once I entered the world of open water swimming, the choice of swimwear became less of an issue. Water is a great leveller and we all battle the same waves. When the water temperature drops, the burkini blends in with the wetsuits.

In 2016, in the aftermath of the short-lived 'Burkini Ban' in France, I had a wild idea to start a swimming group in Australia called the 'Burkini Babes'. I knew a thing or two about feeling policed at the pool, and seeing images of French police officers surrounding a woman because of the clothes she wore, hit a nerve. What began as a political act turned into setting up a bigger group called 'Swim Sisters', formed to create an inclusive environment for *all* women to swim.

Swim Sisters has become a sisterhood of women from all walks of life, ages, backgrounds and fitness abilities, united by a love for the water. The idea flourished, with women keen to be part of an inclusive group for swimmers at all levels: the group attracted new Australians and women who were active in swim squads as children but had taken a pause during their teenage years.

A year later, I became an inadvertent and vocal advocate for 'women only' swimming after giving an interview about the new swimming times introduced at my local pool in Auburn. The women-only times were on Sundays from 3 to 5 p.m. in a 25-metre 'program' pool. Curtains were closed around the pool during the session. In the interview I argued that women's spaces should not be a matter of debate; they were needed to accommodate our diverse local community in one of the most multicultural local government areas in Australia.

The interview became the Auburn pool 'curtain story' and a controversial media item. A headline 'Auburn pool gets swim screen for Muslim women' (Melissa Yeo, *Parramatta Advertiser,* 17 May, 2017) led to a contentious item on the TV show *A Current Affair* and to a divisive swimming instructor inappropriately comparing the initiative to apartheid.

Some men apparently felt offended by not being able to swim for two hours a week in a 25-metre heated program pool. One politician and social commentator created a website called *teardownthatcurtain.com* and asked people to sign a petition in support. Apart from referring to the move to accommodate women swimmers as 'Sharia law', I assume he was being tongue-in-cheek when he asked whether a curtain would next be put up at Bondi Beach. Well, he'd be pleased to know that Bondi is where my Swim Sisters train for our ocean swims, preparing us for qualified surf lifesaving.

If that politician actually cared to listen to women like me, he would understand that beginning my swim journey in a women's pool gave me the confidence to take on ocean water swimming and begin my journey towards becoming a surf lifesaver — to wear red and yellow to protect our beaches. By giving women the comfort of safe, women's swim spaces, we can ensure that the vital survival skills of swimming are shared by all. When you teach a woman to swim, positive water safety is spread within a family and by extension, the entire community.

In my early 20s, I became a 'gym junkie' and trained at a women-only Fernwood gym. During the university holidays, my gym friend, Reem, proposed that we head to the women's rock pool in Coogee, after our morning spin class. From the moment I entered, I was in complete awe of this sanctuary. It was a well-kept secret in my community of Muslim women who made the trek from south-western Sydney, covered from head to toe, carrying their food supplies and making their way to the secluded rocks for a dose of vitamin D and, of course, for the rare opportunity to tan. (Vitamin D deficiency is common among women who wear the hijab and who have limited sun exposure.) I became one of those trekking women.

McIver's is a place where I can let my hair down, literally. It's a place where I press pause on all the noise about my burkini, unwind and lose all notions of time. From the moment I enter the change room with the view of the ocean, everything else pales into insignificance.

My bond to McIver's was further strengthened during my pregnancy. My third trimester coincided with the hottest summer on record. I had an overwhelming urge to immerse myself in the coolness of the water as my baby grew inside me; to ease the ligament soreness in my body and my ever-expanding, swollen feet. I regularly ventured from south-western Sydney to rock pools along the eastern suburbs and kept my one piece swimsuit in my beach bag along with my burkini, just in case I was in the vicinity of McIver's. When I started my maternity leave a week and a half before my due date, I discovered the beauty of quiet afternoon swims.

On the morning of my final antenatal check-up and physiotherapy appointment, I went to relax at the sanctuary that is McIver's and to squeeze in some hypnobirthing practice by the rocks. I sat there with my hair out, breathing in the salty air. I closed my eyes and listened to an audio track of affirmations, telling me that my body was made to do this and that the contractions could be overcome, like surges of the sea. I swam countless laps in the pool, enjoying the priceless feeling of being immersed in the cool water. Within hours of ending my swim, early labour started and my water baby arrived the next day on his due date!

As the last remaining women-only ocean pool in Australia, McIver's speaks to the importance of safe and self-determined spaces for women. Society may have changed significantly since McIver's Baths was built in 1876, but in a society where we continue to grapple with deep-rooted issues such as domestic violence and sexual assault, one thing remains. Women continue to be concerned about their safety. Let's celebrate safe spaces for women in Coogee, Auburn and Roselands and extend them more broadly for all women to enjoy.

*In the throes of a disastrous love affair, author Stephanie Wood writes of the Coogee women's pool, her thinking place.*

# *Fake* [7]

## Stephanie Wood

SUNDAY AFTERNOON. I AM UNSTEADY as I descend the steps to my favourite ocean pool, the ladies' baths, a magnificent Victorian relic cut into sandstone cliffs. Two topless women lean against a railing, their bodies pressed close; one woman caresses the other's lovely tanned arse. A Muslim woman in a neck-to-knee swimsuit, mirroring the black gowns worn here a century or more ago, passes me on the stairs. The water is a glorious bolt of green shot through with shimmering brown-flecked turquoise. An ocean swimmer strokes strongly in the open sea. There are only a few women in the pool and they are standing in a shallow section in the sun, their arms folded and wrapped around their bodies. I stand at the edge, filled with trepidation — it will be cold — then dive. Deep, plunging towards the

---

7   *These extracts are from* Fake *by Stephanie Wood, North Sydney: Penguin Random House, 2019.*

bottom, slicing through the dark frigid water. Then up, towards the surface, with my eyes open, and the shadowy green becomes translucent as I move towards the light and the sky, gasping for breath.

〜

I return to the sea baths. It is spring now and there is a crisp breeze but I plunge in and swim hard. I try to empty my brain and let it fill with the underwater burble, to focus on my stroke, on the reach forward, then pull back, to propel myself through the pool. I think as I swim that I have never seen anything as beautiful as the explosions of bubbles that spring from my hands as they cleave the water — champagne, diamonds, sequins. Under here are ribbons of wriggling light, drifting seaweeds, turban snails gleaming like pearls, a small brown fish with a white spot, a gathering of fussing, flitting fingerlings, the yellow-bellied shell of a dead crab lifting and jerking along the bottom with the water's movement …

〜

One afternoon I return to the ladies' baths, my thinking place. It is grey and drizzly. But for one other woman in a red bathing suit doing slow laps, it is all mine — a rare, delirious joy — and I run down the stairs with the excitement of a child about to swim for the first time since last summer. The stillness is infinite, the water dark and velvety, more jade than turquoise, the sea beyond the pool wall a platinum swathe that blurs into the palest periwinkle blue where it meets the sky.

I could not explain blue before, all the blues, the blue-greens and blue-greys, how they made me feel, the catch in my breath, the multi-tonal thrill of them, but then I found American writer Rebecca Solnit's words on blue — the "color of horizons ... of anything far away ... the color of emotion, the color of solitude and desire, the color of there seen from here, the color of where you are not."[8]

I take some idle strokes, float on my back, porpoise-dive to the bottom, again and again, pursuing glimpses of a tiny fish with electric blue markings that flits and ducks and hides under the rocks. The tide is going out but a rogue wave crashes over the pool wall and over me, and I gasp as the colder water foams like seltzer on my skin. I pause, rest my elbows on the wall, kick my legs behind me and look out towards Wedding Cake Island.

For millennia, Indigenous people swam here in a natural rock pool hugged by a sandstone cliff face. Colonists followed their example and by the 1870s the local council had excavated the rock to deepen the pool, defined it with concrete walls on two sides and segregated it for ladies. (In 1995, the pool was exempted from the state's Anti-Discrimination Act.) I think about how many women before me are likely to have rested their elbows where mine are, laughed as waves crashed over them, and looked out to that low, rocky island with its sea-foam icing. I think, too, about all the women who have found friendships here, or passed on words of kindness or encouragement, as today

---

8   *Rebecca Solnit,* A Field Guide to Getting Lost, *Canongate, 2017, p. 29, North Sydney: Penguin 2006.*

a group of older women did to me as we crossed paths at the entrance. "The water is beautiful," said one, and her friends nodded enthusiastically. So beautiful they just had to share the good news with a stranger. There is here a sense of gentle continuity. I feel I am one of an unbroken chain of women who have, over generations, come to the pool seeking inspiration or motivation or answers; who have brought fears and worries, about love or health or money or who knows what else; who have come to cleanse themselves of anger or pain or trauma, or to expel their demons And I wonder how many women have felt their troubles soften, even dissolve, in this water, and have returned to the world feeling lighter.

I look again at Wedding Cake Island and think about the concept of human damage. I have sometimes been susceptible to the idea that I am damaged. I have thought that my wounds must be as evident as if I had just yesterday been punched in the eye. But I know now that this thinking is absurd. If I turn my back on the iconic little island, beaten and battered by the sea for aeons, I come face to face with the sandstone cliff that forms the two walls of the pool. The sandstone is layered with colour — tan, pink, cream, ochre — and over the centuries has been contoured by the wind and sand. We do not think of it as damaged, we look at it and think it is lovely.

So, too, is a life, a character, shaped and variegated and enriched in the wild moments and the storms, by difficulties and mistakes, misfortunes and, humiliations, tragedies and traumas. I am not the person I was before. I don't want to be the person I was before. I like myself now better than I ever did. I like the bruises, the sore sad spots and the scars. I treasure them as precious spoils of war, evidence that I fell over, then got back up again, that I fought wild beasts — including the beast that is my brain — and won. That I am strong, that I can roar.

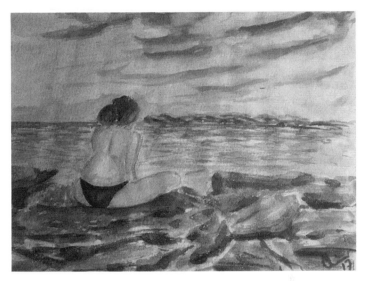

*Looking to Wedding Cake Island*
Watercolour by Clarissa de Castro Lima

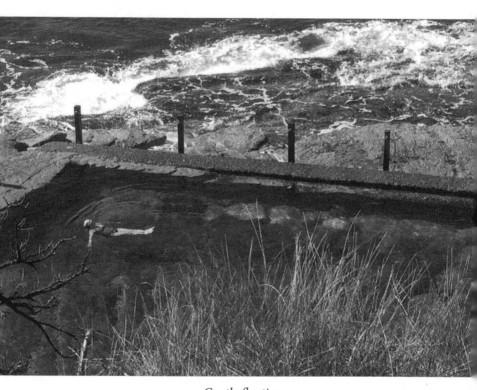

*Gently floating*
Photograph by Wendy Assinder

*Helen Pringle considers the complexities of asserting women's right of exclusive access to (some) public spaces.*

# Leave These Women Alone ...

## Helen Pringle

AS A YOUNG GIRL, I travelled great distances by car with my family. We made frequent toilet stops, with our parents regularly asking us, "Are you comfortable?" or "Do you need to go?" We rarely managed to synchronise our need 'to go', and often had to stop more times than there were rest areas along the way. My father would stop the car at the side of the road and we 'went' between back and front doors, opened to screen us from the view of passing cars. Whether at rest area toilets or at the roadside, my parents would urge my sisters and me to "Be careful," although my brothers did not seem to get a similar caution.

When we did go to public toilets, the reason for this caution became clear. On the wall of the toilet, there was often a drawing of a semi-erect penis and testicles, with droplets from one end. These drawings lacked captions; their little readers were left to work out the meaning for themselves.

This drawing was like the signature of a tomcat spraying its territorial domain — in the women's toilet. But it was also a sign to all girls that we were never free from being looked at, even in our more vulnerable moments. Our space was never truly ours. Even in territory marked 'Female' or 'Ladies', we ventured there on men's terms, their forbearance.

There are few places of shelter or seclusion for women to gather: our world is truly a 'man's world'. One place, however, is McIver's Ladies Baths in a corner of Coogee, where I live. McIver's is not merely a baths or pool, although swimming is the explicit purpose of the little clearing on the cliff. The 'space' of McIver's includes rocks and a patch of grass, with stairs leading up and down from the change room and the office of the women who are its unobtrusive guardians. For women, McIver's offers a place of seclusion and shelter, not only from the wearying and constant reminder of our corporeal 'flaws' ('Are you beach body ready?' as an infamous weight-loss advertisement on the London Tube asked in 2015) but just from being stared at, pawed at by the eyes of strangers as well as familiars.

Kandy James has written of the unsettling effects on girls of experiencing themselves as objects that are stared at, and of the measures that girls take in such circumstances to make themselves unavailable, even invisible — for example, by not going to pools or beaches at all. The Australian beach for many young girls is less a place of peaceful enjoyment of swimming and other leisure activities and more like a battleground, a field of gazes, on which questions of our composure as women and our freedom as a sex are fought out.

McIver's was managed from 1922 by the Randwick and Coogee Ladies Amateur Swimming Club (now the Randwick & Coogee Ladies Swimming Association) for Randwick Council, which leases the land from the Crown. The 'Ladies' have somehow managed to absent women from male surveillance for 100 years. Paradoxically, the first serious threat to the seclusion of McIver's came after the passing of the 1977 NSW Anti-Discrimination Act, which provides redress for discriminatory acts in various contexts and supports equal opportunity, across a variety of grounds, including sex.

In December 1992, Leon Wolk, a resident of Coogee, wrote to the NSW Anti-Discrimination Board, drawing attention to a sign at the entrance to McIver's Baths which said 'Ladies and Children's Pool'. Wolk asked, "Is this permissible? If it is permissible, why? Should it not be permissible, what is necessary to have this sign removed?" (*Wolk v Randwick City Council* 1995, §92–721).

McIver's policy of excluding men had consisted largely of unspoken undertakings and mutual understandings. Mr Wolk's complaint was that this was unlawful, and fostered inequality more generally. In January 1993, Randwick Council responded by passing a unanimous motion in support of the pool being retained for 'the exclusive use' of women and boys under 13 years of age. A rowdy group of women attended the Council meeting to make their thoughts and feelings known.

In March 1995, in response to an application made under the §126A 'special needs programs and activities' provision of the Anti-Discrimination Act, the then Minister for Local

Government, Ted Pickering, granted McIver's Ladies Baths a permanent exemption from discrimination provisions. The rationale was that the 'women only' policy was a measure to ensure equal or improved access to members of groups subjected to unlawful discrimination in regard to facilities, services and opportunities. The 'special needs' of women were the enabling of access for women with disabilities or Muslim women and girls, as well as the privacy, safety and sociability needs of women more generally. Such concerns were voiced by representations to the Minister by women's groups, and in surveys of users of the pool by the Kingsford Legal Centre.

Mr Wolk's complaint was further addressed by the Equal Opportunity Tribunal after conciliation efforts with the Council faltered. In March 1995, the Tribunal found that Mr Wolk's case failed on the basis that the issue in hand was not a discriminatory 'provision of goods and services' but rather 'access' to a place, and that Mr Wolk's initial allegations should be dismissed as 'frivolous or vexatious'.

Kurt Iveson (2007) has explored this dispute about access to McIver's Baths within the wider context of the ways in which some forms of exclusion, or protection of seclusion, can work not to weaken public solidarity and the assurance of equal justice, but to nurture forms of conviviality (or in this case, perhaps sorority) across other differences such as age, class and status, race and ethnicity, and religion. In other words, excluding men from McIver's was not a simple matter of exclusion, but of developing valuable civic solidarities among women. The dispute was not merely about leisure activities but, in some sense at least, about equal opportunities for meaningful civic participation; the case for 'women only' access was not just for the protection of women but to enhance their civic standing.

Women surveyed about the issue by the Kingsford Legal Centre made frequent mention of McIver's as a shelter. Pat Richardson portrayed the scene on the Coogee rocks in 1992:

> It was a glorious day. We ladies sat around like happy sea lions, sunbaked topless, swam unmolested and unstared at. Our stretch marks bothered no-one. Our Caesareans, our bulges, our cellulite, our pregnancies were all our own. Fifteen-stone mermaids like me could frolic, unsneered at by fat-gutted males with balding pates. In fact, I could feel a poem coming on (Richardson, 1992, p. 237).

Other women spoke of the question of composure, in terms of how the women-only setting of McIver's permitted them to compose themselves on their own terms in a space of their own:

> With just women and small children, it is quiet, peaceful and safe. There are not many places you can go without being subjected to the loud showing-off of young men. It is such a small pool that the presence of men would take up the entire space (quoted in Iveson, 2007, p. 199).

Some women referred to the way the presence of men was disturbing to the purpose of the baths. For example, Ms Fran Blackbourne, 28, said she would stop coming if men moved in:

> I'm fairly self-conscious about my body and I don't feel comfortable being stared at … There's an amazing feeling to this place, with no men strutting their bodies and doing

that 'in your face' sexual thing. And mothers can bring their kids here without worrying about who they are talking to (in Moore and Freeman, 2000).

Lorna Mobbs, one of the McIver's guardians, noted, "It's the only pool in Sydney where you don't have to put up with men." Mrs Mobbs did, however, mention that men had tried to "burn us out," had vandalised the pool, and in one case had "drilled a hole in the change room wall to peep at the women inside" (in Connell, 1993, p. 9).

Not having 'to put up with men' also enabled women to conduct their lives in a different way. It is striking that standard pictures of women swimming in the rock pool portray them as gently floating on their backs rather than doing more stereotypically masculine water activities like vigorous laps or bombing, activities dissonant with the gentleness of the pool and the space in which it is set.

Much more recently, claims of discrimination have again been made against the pool: in this case, discrimination on the grounds of transgender status. In December 2010, for example, a person of masculine appearance came to the pool area with two female companions who claimed that their friend was undertaking hormone therapy. The appearance of the bare-chested person caused consternation among Muslim girls in the pool, who left, and a report was made to the lifesavers (in Pitt, 2010).

In 2021, this question was raised again, but with more voices. McIver's responded that trans women *were* allowed entry to the space of the pool, but only those who had undergone gender reassignment surgery.

In response, the University of Sydney Women's

Collective published a statement (with Content Warnings for "transphobia, suicide, sexual violence" to condemn this policy as "an act of public and violent transphobia." The Collective demanded a change in policy as well as a public apology. The statement claimed that "Trans women need safe leisure spaces such as the Ladies Baths more than cisgender (*sic*) women do, as they face a higher risk of gendered violence." The Collective's post on Facebook was accompanied by selfies of women students sitting in empty bathtubs.

A campaign calling to 'Let them swim' was launched. This was odd in that the right to swim was not in dispute, only the right to enter and use a particular area designated for the use of women and children only.

Some of the opposition to McIver's policy was based on invoking the mythic, even magical, qualities of water and the benefits of communing with it. This, again, was not in contention. There is water, no end of water, in Coogee and along the Sydney coastline. And there are many other pools, with rocks and patches of grass, and change rooms.

To understand the claim of trans women to the right to enter women-only spaces like McIver's is not a simple matter. Rather, it is to grapple with very difficult questions of discrimination, equality and public life. In the 'provision of goods and services', the comparison is made with a similarly placed and non-gendered 'person'. That is, anti-discrimination measures do not require that we treat a person without any regard to gender, but rather with regard to enabling their equal enjoyment of the world. It is not a harm to regulate access to a place, even one of such magic and light as McIver's, if enough and as much enjoyment can be provided elsewhere.

Women are entitled to space, and time to enjoy life in our own way and with respect to our own heritage, customs, mores and traditions, *as* women — especially in terms of developing our rich history of attachment, loyalty and even love for social relations in a place of great and simple beauty.

During the 1995 legal challenge to access to McIver's, *The Sydney Morning Herald* editorialised in support of keeping access to the pool for women only. "Leave these women alone," the editorial writer pleaded. This remains a timely injunction: leave them alone to develop in their own time and space, in concert and conviviality with other women, without intrusion.

## References

Anti-Discrimination Act 1977 (NSW). <https://www.legislation.nsw.gov.au/view/whole/html/inforce/current/act-1977-048>.

Connell, Jennifer. 27 December 1993. 'Pool'. *The Sydney Morning Herald.*

Iveson, Kurt. 2007. 'Justifying exclusion: Keeping men out of the Ladies' Baths, Sydney'. Chapter 7 in *Publics and the City.* Oxford: Blackwell.

James, Kandy. 2000. 'You can feel them looking at you: The experiences of adolescent girls at swimming pools'. *Journal of Leisure Research* Vol. 32 Issue 2, pp. 262–280.

Minister for Local Government and Cooperatives [Edward Phillip Pickering]. 3 March 1995. *Certification under Section 126A of the Anti-Discrimination Act 1977.*

Moore, Matthew and Jane Freeman. 17 January 1995. 'Equality makes waves where women seek still waters'. *The Sydney Morning Herald.*

Pitt, Helen. 11 December 2010. 'Martha or Arthur? Cossies in a twist at ladies-only baths'. *The Sydney Morning Herald.*

Richardson, Pat. 1992. *Belle on a Broomstick*. Sydney: Gum Leaf Press.

*The Sydney Morning Herald*. 18 January 1995. Editorial: 'Leave these women alone'.

University of Sydney Women's Collective. 2021. 'Public statement on the McIver Ladies Baths transphobic entry policy'.

*Wolk v Randwick City Council* (1995) EOC §92–721.

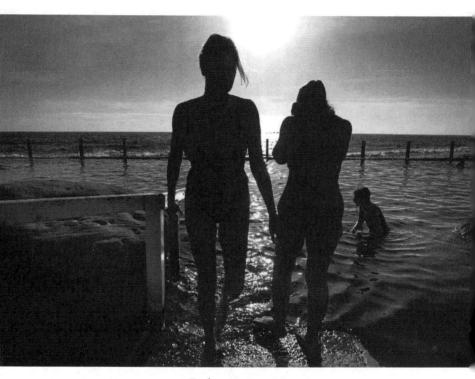

*Early morning swim*
Photograph by Kate Geraghty, *Sydney Morning Herald*

*Living with Ehlers-Danlos syndrome, Dominique Pile finds that swimming becomes an essential part of her life.*

# Second Skin

## Dominique Pile

AT THE AGE OF 13, my relationship with pools changed from casual indulgence to quiet commitment when my parents decided that swimming was the only sport I should continue to do in my high school years.

I have Ehlers-Danlos syndrome, a genetic disorder which affects my connective tissue, joints and blood vessels. Nowadays, there's a large body of research into this hereditary condition but back in the 1970s, we just called it 'stretchy skin'. It gave me two party tricks to impress my young friends: double jointed thumbs that arch dramatically into a hitchhiking position and elastic skin that they could stretch down from my straightened elbows like glutinous pizza dough. Simultaneously repugnant and fascinating.

The downside of my skin is that when I fall on hard surfaces, it tears like cellophane and bruises like a rotten peach. By age 13, I had the scars to prove it.

Not being able to participate in basketball or tennis with my friends made me feel like the odd one out, but secretly I loved the solitude of the pool and the softness of the water. It was also a genuine relief not to have to play hockey. During my teenage years, fresh and saltwater pools became my playground, my refuge, my solace; swimming was the one physical activity I thought I could possibly excel at. But competition was never a real driver and swimming was far more to me than just a sport.

The water understood my body. It too has elastic properties. It held my feet, my scarred knees, my bruised legs, my arms and my torso with perfect assurance and transformed a body that was a liability on land into that of a water sprite. I really did feel like a fish in water.

More than 40 years later, water is still my protective layer and swimming has become my second skin. It is the aquatic metronome to my life — the experiential touchstone. Staccato skinny dips with boys as a self-conscious 16-year-old at Paradise Beach; languid swims in my 30s in the crystal waters of Crete; stress-busting laps before work in my 40s; an impromptu dip at the Coogee women's pool in middle age.

A regular dip in waterholes, pools, rivers, dams, lakes or oceans has always brought my mind back into my body and my body back to life — and more. Swimming in different places also provides a window into the personality and habits of the locals. In Portugal, I watched admiring locals encircle a fit-looking silver fox as he emerged from the brisk water and made his way up the beach. Who was this affable man smiling in selfies with children and kissing men and women on both cheeks? In 'Portugenglish', I asked one of his fans, "Es un actor famoso"? "Não, ele é o Presidente"! he replied. It was Marcelo Nuno Duarte Rebelo de Sous, the President of Portugal, himself an avid swimmer.

In the early 1990s, I was a regular at the Piscine Pontoise in the Latin Quarter of Paris; a beautiful Art Deco pool, built in 1934. It was here that director, Krzysztof Kieslowski filmed Juliette Binoche's character, processing her grief and anger as she swims in his meditative masterpiece, *Three Colours: Blue*. At the time, the walls of the pool were a light sky blue, the doors to the individual changing cabins a deep cobalt blue. The decor was cool and ordered and elegant but, in the water, it was mayhem. Parisians had yet to discover the system of swimming up and down in a clockwise manner or creating separate lanes to stop serious lappers and playful splashers from colliding. Perhaps international visitors had a word with the Piscine's management, but progress has been made and there is order now.

In the mid-90s and early 2000s, the silky, brown water of the Ladies' Pond on Hampstead Heath was my delight in summer and my dare in winter. The women-only pond is located in a secluded spot on the heath. Self-assured young women sunbaked bare-breasted, flirting furtively with their girlfriends amongst the 'straights' picnicking on the grass. Lesbian Londoners were on the loose in a seductively restrained kind of way and the bucolic atmosphere of the pond made me feel as if I were in a Jane Austen novel with an updated cast of characters. I was the shy one.

After 17 years abroad, I returned to Sydney in 2005 and found it hard to reacclimatise. In my efforts to knit an authentic life for myself back home, swimming proved a golden thread. I discovered the delights of Clovelly: an inlet with a reef that feels more like an aquarium than an ocean beach. And on one unbearably hot Saturday night in 2016, I finally entered the inner sanctum of Coogee women's pool to engage in an illicit activity that's a highlight in my calendar of aquatic memories.

2016 was a record-breaking summer in NSW, a meteorological state of affairs that has largely become the norm for our summers now, thanks to climate change. My partner and our two good friends had finished dinner at a local restaurant and wandered out onto the Coogee promenade. The humidity was cloying. It was too hot to sleep and the wine had unlocked our desire for adventure. There was nothing for it but a skinny dip in the pool …

As we made our way down the steep steps in the dark, I could feel the elements penetrating my senses: warm air, cool rock, seawater, the smell of salt, the sound of waves.

At the base of the cliff, the intimate, well-worn rock pool revealed itself to us in the moonlight, looking much as it might have over 150 years ago when women's lives were as restricted as their corseted bodies. How liberating it must have felt for women in the 1830s to unfasten their heavy, tight clothing and let the water support their bodies as they bathed — and later, learned to swim.

That night we giggled at our mischievous transgression as we stripped off and slipped into the cooling water, breaking its perfect surface and cheekily disturbing its peace. In return, the pool restored order to our over-heated bodies and enveloped us in its calm. I felt privileged to have been given such a special introduction to this aquatic refuge, hiding in plain sight. The Baths still have an air of secrecy about them and I had finally joined those in the know.

The tableau remains vivid: four mature women feeling like water nymphs, revelling in our waywardness as we floated around the pool laughing with our tits proudly up. I realise now that I'm no longer the only 'stretchy' one in the pool. I couldn't be more at home in my second skin.

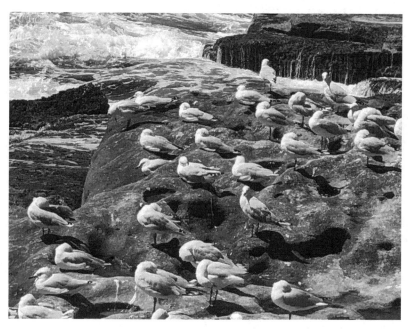

*Gulls on the McIver's rocks*
Photograph by Wendy Assinder

*Except during high summer, Louise Sprinkle is a respectable mother and grandmother.*

# Mrs Sprinkle's Moonlight Madness

## Louise P. Sprinkle

I WAS NEW TO THE EASTERN SUBURBS when I discovered the women's pool. To my delight, I found a community of like-minded mature mermaids and water babes. The ocean holds all kinds of magical and healing elixirs, which never fail to wash away my blues.

I could not have imagined just how much my life would be changed by the pool. The women were so welcoming, and we all laughed and sometimes shared our stories (of divorce, parenting, affairs, recalcitrant children and demanding grandchildren), while playfully splashing in the waves like dolphins, then undertaking serious laps in our caps.

One woman in particular caught my attention. It started with laughter and jokes, but I felt a connection on a level that was new to me. As the days turned to weeks we sometimes met for a dusk swim, watched the horizon turn pink, and had a drink or picnic. Our visits got later and later, and soon we were swimming nude by moonlight! What would my daughters think, if they could see me now?

I began to realise quite how much (and how!) I wanted this woman at the pool. After more nocturnal swimming in the heat of summer and sitting on the grass afterwards, talking in the night air, we became lovers. Never having been with a woman in this way before, I was captivated by how natural and exciting it felt. What an adventure.

One night, after a quick dip, we were alone at the pool, and somehow ended up in one of the outdoor change cubicles, exploring more than its three close walls, narrow slatted bench, and bolted wooden door. Mid-excitement, we heard a deep cough, unmistakably emanating from a man. Through a crack in the wooden door, we could see the light of the man's cigarette, and hear him swigging from a bottle. He was sitting with his back to us, less than a metre away. We held each other, hearts pounding, and prayed we would each stay quiet — no laughing, sneezing, or heavy breathing!

It took an eternity for Mr Man to finish his cigarette. He wasn't going anywhere. I really hoped he hadn't planned to meet someone else here and use one of these cubicles himself! (I had heard that the early morning lady swimmers had not infrequently found condoms on the lawn.) Eventually, he coughed again, cleared his throat, then stood up, tossed his bottle into the bushes, and sauntered up the path. Phew. We rocked with relief and spluttered our suppressed sniggers into each other's necks.

That was our last swim of summer. Things change. They always do. But whenever I go back to the pool these days, sometimes with my grandchildren, I try to use that same change cubicle, and joyfully reflect on the strong, independent, sensual woman I have become. And who knows what next summer will bring?

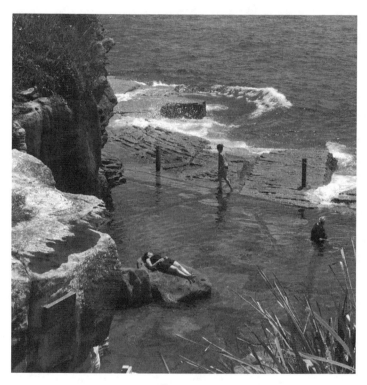

*Recovery*
Photograph by Tracy Grujovic

*Maddy Proud writes about recovery from playing professional netball and her joy at discovering the women's pool as a place for physical and emotional recuperation.*

# Recovery

## Maddy Proud

HOW WOULD THE SEDATE LADIES at the serene and peaceful McIver's Ladies Baths react to 12 shrieking netballers descending on the pool for a recovery session? I think they'd cope. Unlike most 'secret societies', these women actually seem to take pleasure in others enjoying the pool. They are the first to offer a grand tour for newcomers and although most workers are volunteers, they sell the place as if they're pocketing a hefty commission.

I arrived in Sydney from Adelaide at the end of 2016, ready for a new journey with the NSW Swifts in the Suncorp Super Netball competition. And while things on the court were going swimmingly (no pun intended), I struggled during my first few years living so far from the beach. Growing up, my two brothers and I had the luxury of having a pool in our backyard *and* the beach at the end of the street. I'd taken this for granted and it wasn't until I made the move to the big smoke that I realised just how much I missed it. It didn't take me long to get used to hopping in the car, turning up my favourite Taylor Swift album and making my way through the traffic to one of Sydney's many stunning beaches. I immediately fell in love with the beach culture of Sydney. I loved how every beach in each area was so different and diverse and had its own set of rules and way of life. I loved the rivalries between the east and the north (and some would say the south). And gee, did I love the ocean pools. Swimming pool and the ocean. It combined two of my favourite things in the world and suddenly I understood why everyone raved about the harbour city and everything it had to offer.

Swimming is the ultimate relief. There is no better feeling than diving into the cool water on a hot day and feeling it rush past your face. And while the pool in the backyard of my current Canada Bay oasis has helped keep me cool during the prolonged summer heatwaves, it doesn't quite have the same tranquillity as the McIver's women's pool at Coogee. The first day I weaved my way down the steps, placed my belongings on a semi-submerged rock and dived into the crisp, cool water, I knew it would become my recovery destination of choice. I was also determined to turn the Coogee pool regulars into Swifts fans and convince them to trek it to the west to watch us play.

"Alright girls, time for ice baths," is one of the most haunting phrases you can hear after a training session. Netball is a gruelling sport, particularly hard on your joints. I've torn cartilage in both of my knees and I underwent a knee reconstruction 18 months ago, so to say recovery is an important part of my training regime is an understatement. I've played at the professional level for almost ten years now, and I no longer dread the post-match recovery sessions if it means I manage to do them in Coogee.

Recovery methods have evolved throughout the years, from hot and cold showers, ice baths, recovery boots and compression — to new cutting-edge technologies, each claiming to reap the benefits faster than any other. But the one constant has been active recovery in the water. There is no substitute for wading through the cool water or doing a gentle freestyle to loosen your tired and sore limbs. No matter how cold the ocean is, the scenery and ambience can make you *feel* as if it's ten degrees warmer. It is certainly less likely to evoke the collective shrieks of 12 girls than a freezing ice bath.

Sometimes the mental recovery is just as, if not more, important than the physical. Sport can be cruel and after a tough loss, a hard session or a painful injury, your mind needs to be cleared just as much as your body. That's where McIver's shines again. Somehow your limbs *and* your mind feel lighter when the sun is on your face and you are nestled among the rockpools surrounding the baths. With bustling Coogee beach within sight, the juxtaposition between the herds of beachgoers fighting for a spot on the sand and the almost eerie peacefulness of the baths is special. You just can't help but feel happy.

I'd like to think it gives me a competitive advantage, too. I sleep more deeply on a Sunday night and wake fresher on a Monday morning after an afternoon at the baths. My mind is sharper, my legs are nimbler and the week ahead feels like a new opportunity rather than a repeat of the one before. I've begged our coaches to let the entire team do a recovery session at McIver's, knowing that if we can all feel the same way as I do on a Monday morning, it could be just what we need to take home the trophy at the end of the year.

I can picture it now: Sam, our Trinidadian goal shooter, squealing as we force her into the water, floaties in hand. Sarah, a self-proclaimed 'sinker', slipping on her flippers in the hope that they will keep her afloat; water-baby Loz diving straight in and not coming up for air until she's at the other end of the pool. Gossip about dating lives will be interspersed with game debriefs and complaints of poor umpiring decisions until suddenly a quiet calmness will overcome the group and the baths will work their magic. I'm not a meditator but the feeling amongst the team will be as if we are in a trance. And then the spell will be broken, splashes will be exchanged and the squeals will get louder. But tranquillity doesn't always mean silence, does it? I hope the ladies don't think so, anyway. Hopefully, some free tickets and a Swifts one-piece cozzie will convince them.

*A regular morning swimmer, Deborah deals with fear and a moment of celebrity at the pool. The celebrity status fades but the pleasure of the pool remains.*

# Trouble in Paradise

## Deborah Kneeshaw

A GLORIOUS WINTER DAY. Bright sunlight making rainbows in crystal clear water. Post-swim, I warm myself on the rocks. I'm at the wonderful women's pool and — for once — I have it all to myself. Bliss.

Yet, somehow, I feel anxious. A niggle tells me that something is not right. Is it fear? Maybe it's because I am reading a book by Wayne Dyer, an American self-help guru. "Change your thoughts," he says. "Don't give in to fear." Got it, Wayne. But my body is not buying it.

I look up and catch sight of a man. He shouldn't be here. He clocks my gaze and springs into the bushes. He's big. Way bigger than I am. I watch his baseball cap bobbing around in the foliage as he makes his way up the bank, secreting himself in the undergrowth above the stairs to the exit — my only way out. I look around. It's just me and him. I'm trapped.

What to do? B-R-E-A-T-H-E. And dial 000. Emergency. I find my phone and do it. I dial. My heart is beating fast. Adrenaline. Fight or flight.

I determine not to move from my rock and the relative safety of being visible from the coastal walk above. We sit it out. He lurks, hidden, he thinks. I breathe deeply. I'm trying, Wayne, I'm trying.

The stand-off, perhaps ten minutes — but it seems longer — is interrupted by two policewomen who appear on the far side of the baths, above the pool. They see me and I gesture frantically to them as they make their way down to me.

Then, just like a scripted TV drama, it's action stations. He makes a dash across the grounds behind the police and our two heroines turn and chase him. He dives into the dense bushes above the pool and they stop. A moment of silence. Then horror! He seems to be spat out. I tentatively move towards the pool and recoil as I see him on the rocks, metres below. He doesn't move.

The tide is coming in and a wave washes over him. A bigger wave pulls him towards the roiling ocean. He groans and lies there, helpless, holding his leg.

Holy shit, I think. I'm going to be responsible for someone drowning.

There is no such empathy from the police officers. They head down to the pool and edge their way around it. They climb onto the adjacent rocks and, seemingly impervious to his injuries, haul him back from the waves. I watch, conflicted, as he is escorted, more like dragged, up the pool stairs to the waiting paddy-wagon. He is moaning and clutching his leg (a fracture, I suspect). Then it's over and I can't quite process what has happened. It doesn't stop me from thinking I wouldn't want to mess with those women police officers.

Later, we mused that the baseball-capped intruder may well have been the infamous 'wanker' who had been hanging around for months, intimidating swimmers and sunbathers at the women's pool. We certainly didn't see him again.

For a while after the drama, I became a minor celebrity at the pool. My welcome was assured. The pool quietly returned to being a safe place but I never returned to Wayne Dyer. There may be times when we need to ignore or push through our fears but there are other times when fear deserves our full attention.

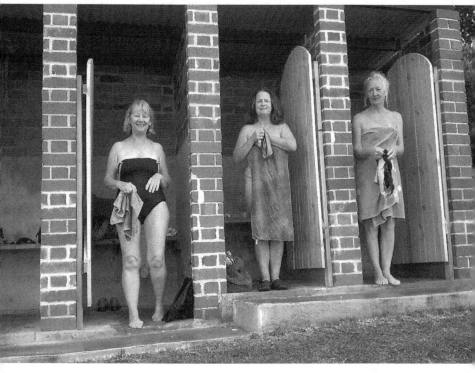

*In the wooden change sheds*
Photograph by Wendy Freeman

*A long-time pool user, Rhonda Fadden reflects on her 40 years of visiting the women's pool.*

# A Small Sense of Freedom

## Rhonda Fadden

MY FIRST VISITS TO THE WOMEN'S POOL were in the 80s. That was before the pool became widely-known and sometimes, I had the whole pool to myself. Perhaps because I swam early and late, and during the off peak seasons. For me, the autumn mornings were, and still are, particularly good.

The Randwick and Coogee Ladies Amateur Swimming Club ran the McIver's Baths — we just it called the women's pool. It was an enjoyable women-only social space. The pool and the areas around it felt like they had been used and protected by many women over many decades, and the clubhouse had the feel of a warm, well-loved women's place.

Members met regularly at the clubhouse, now called the office. As I went past the door, I could see, but mostly hear, a group of older women chatting, joking, playing cards and having morning tea or lunch. I know there was a

Thursday Married Ladies Club then. I think they still meet on Thursdays.

In those years, there wasn't a lot of engagement between club members and visitors; we tossed our 20 cents in a bin inside the front door with a nod and a smile. I was aware that members kept an eye out for any problems and were happy to answer queries about the weather, the tides and the likelihood of bluebottles, but I sensed they were not there to serve or to supervise closely. Rather, they gave the impression that they were there to enjoy their seclusion and their obvious camaraderie. I had no idea then just how much voluntary work they did — the cleaning, removing rubbish, and getting leaky taps and toilets fixed, along with their overall care and stewardship of the pool. In the late 80s the club members didn't like women removing their bikini tops. It seemed the least I could do, to respectfully follow their rules and requests.

I went to the pool to improve my fitness, to enjoy a quiet swim and for the occasional chats. But mostly I went there for the women-only space, the gently respectful atmosphere, and for the pool itself. On one of my first visits a pod of dolphins swam south between the pool and Wedding Cake Island. Not such an unusual event on this part of the coast, but I'd rarely seen them so near, leaping together with the sun shining on their backs. Since then I've seen a few repeat performances. Wildness, so close by.

I liked the wooden change sheds, in a row above the outdoor shower. They reminded me of old sheds at the beaches and creeks of my childhood. They face the ocean, so you can dress and undress with the door open, looking out to sea. Why does that feel so good? A small sense of freedom.

One day, in my first year at the pool, the tranquillity was shattered. A woman near me started screaming, clutching her towel around her and pointing up the hill. Under the trees, but not out of sight, there was a man, pants around his ankles, masturbating. I yelled out, others did too. He scrabbled and tripped his way up the hill to our jeering. On my way out, I told the women in the clubhouse, thinking they would need to report it — to the local council? the police? "Hmm, that happens," one said. They weren't indifferent, but they sounded inured. Clearly, such intrusions were not uncommon.

The grounds were re-landscaped a few years later, after lobbying from the club. Among the improvements, the council built a high, non-see-through fence at the top of the site and rebuilt the sunbathing area with a higher wall, to protect the privacy of sunseekers. They also levelled out a few of the sloping and rough areas, making them more comfortable for lying around, reading and chatting.

Even with those changes, much of the pool area is steep and uneven, and the space is physically inaccessible for some women and a challenge for others. It is a tumbling-down-the-cliff area, partly natural, irregular and rocky, with native and exotic plants and grassy patches and the pool — down and down sets of irregular stairs.

Like other sea pools on the coast, the women's pool can be a surprisingly good spot to snorkel: fun to show children and visiting friends the fish, the small crabs in the crannies of rocky walls, the occasional octopus and sometimes nudibranchs. The sea hares on the rock shelves are slimy-looking, but are very efficient cleaners of mossy rocks. In late summer, when the warm current has come to Sydney, there can be juvenile tropical fish, often absurdly miniature versions of black, white and yellow patterned butterfly fish.

One day in 1995 the clubhouse was abuzz — with a bigger crowd, empty bottles of Great Western bubbly and plates with leftover lamingtons and cakes. The club was celebrating the decision of the Equal Opportunity Tribunal to dismiss a complaint that, in being refused access to McIver's Baths, a man had been discriminated against on the ground of his sex.

The complaint was first made in 1994 against Randwick Council, which leases the baths from the NSW Government — in those years, from the Department of Conservation and Land Management. The club applied for, and was granted, leave to be joined as a third party to the inquiry and Kingsford Legal Centre appeared on their behalf.

The club's campaign was a focal point for local and other Sydney women who used the pool. Support also came from women who hadn't swum at the pool, but believed it should continue as a women only space, and the campaign developed quickly as a broader women's issue. I remember the big turnout at a Randwick Council meeting and the wide diversity of women who were involved. There had been earlier challenges to the pool's exclusive use by women. In 1946 an attempt to include men was thwarted by the local Brigidine Convent's swimming nuns, who successfully asserted their need for the pool to remain open for women only.

I loved swimming in the pool at night. It always felt safe to me, even when I was there alone. There was a delicious sense of personal freedom in a secret haven so close to the big city, and it was magical in the moonlight. One night I arrived at about 10 p.m., anticipating a solo swim. I came to a halt outside the clubhouse that looks over the pool. Two men were sitting on the edge of the pool, quietly chatting. If I'd asked them to leave, they probably would have gone without fuss, but I couldn't risk it. I left feeling anger and a sad loss of autonomy and safety. I haven't swum there at night since then.

The popularity of the pool has increased over the years. That, along with new health and safety regulations, has increased the need for more organised supervision. In 2017, a friend suggested I help out, so I joined the volunteer group. Volunteers wore a yellow shirt and floppy hat, both emblazoned with the pool's name, so that we stood out. I like to think this enhanced my authority, but I wonder. We collected the entry fee, answered questions, told recalcitrants to stop smoking, looked for lost property, helped anyone with a problem, and chatted.

I enjoyed learning the ropes from long-term volunteers, and hearing stories of the history of the club and the pool. There were very few real problems. Most of the women who visited were relaxed and courteous and, with experienced older hands and trained volunteers and staff, the daily routines and occasional dramas were managed with good cheer and professionalism.

Now, visitor numbers can reach peak capacity on hot summer days and entry has to be monitored and limited to the maximum allowable numbers. A queue can extend from the front gate down the hill, with women waiting for someone to leave before they can enter. Even with the physical limitations of the site, and the occasional restrictions on numbers, it's obvious that many women want a pool and space for women only. There are still very few options in Sydney and perhaps it is time for coastal councils to provide some new, ocean swimming spaces for women? It would be a popular move, I'm sure. And it would take some of the increasing pressure off McIver's as the only ocean pool dedicated to women and their safety.

Since my first visits almost 40 years ago, I see a much wider diversity of women visiting the pool. Women who once contributed to its management have come and gone, and the smaller more intimate community has evolved too. I still enjoy being there, in the quieter times, but I've moved on from being involved in the organisation. I'm happy — and hopeful — about leaving it to a younger generation of women and newer users to ensure McIver's remains this unique, welcoming, and safe women's place.

*As a relatively new Coogee resident, Belinda Buchan discovers that it's never too soon to take your children to the women's pool.*

# They Start Them Young at the Women's Pool

## Belinda Buchan

SOME TIME AGO I agreed to let my two and four-year-old daughters spend time at McIver's Ladies Baths while their grandmother was on volunteer duty. I was only slightly concerned, mainly about her tolerance levels, rather than their safety. When I went to collect them, the four-year-old was 'helping' the volunteers by taking the $2 coins from the women coming down the entry stairs and the two-year-old was raiding the lolly jar on the table in the club room. Their grandmother seemed unconcerned.

I came back a few weeks later with the girls who were excited they were going again to the women's pool. "Can I get the money?" "Will there be treats?"

It was a hot March morning, perfect for a mother and daughter outing, and as I walked down the path towards the clubhouse, daughters and beach bags in tow, I remember thinking, please let this go smoothly. I was not a Coogee native and had not previously been to the pool for a swim, and certainly not with two small children. I still saw myself as a 'new' mother and was afraid that, at best, the girls would have tantrums and, at worst, that one of them would fall in the water and drown.

It did not go smoothly.

Tossing my coin in the bucket, while corralling the girls, my first impressions were of women basking in the sun, reading books, talking to their friends. They looked *so* carefree and relaxed. Freedom, I thought. I will get there again one day. There will be time in the future for me to come back for this.

The women gave warm, encouraging smiles as I moved further into the grounds. I had heard that the pool was great for people-watching. As a tired and self-conscious mother, trying to juggle a bag, packed with too many unnecessary items, and battling to keep one daughter on her hip and a toddler from face-planting on the uneven stairs, I felt I must have provided an interesting spectacle.

I tried to choose a spot away from people, so as not to disturb them with my novice mothering and I began preparation for the pool. "Let's put your floaties on, shall we?" Floaties went on. Floaties were pulled off. "Now, let's stop the sun making your cheeks red". The sunscreen scramble. It's in their eyes, it's in my eyes. It's barely on their cheeks. They complain loudly. I apologise to those around. "Keep your hats on, I whisper!" Hats go on, oh no — one hat off and blowing away. I rush to recover it, apologising to the reclining women whom I disturb on the way. I tell myself it will all be worth it once we enter the water.

I pick up the younger one (with hat on) and walk gingerly down the stairs, hand in hand with the four-year-old (hat off, but sunscreen on). Sun on our faces and water glistening; the turquoise hue reminds me of Greece and Italy. Women of all ages, shapes and sizes are chatting, meditating, floating or swimming in the pool, without any interruptions from noisy little ones. I was aware of my presence and of the children, afraid that their squeals would cause other women around me to judge my parenting, or scold me for disrupting the peace of the pool. But the opposite happened.

I was balancing precariously on the steps when an older woman offered to hold the younger child; the four-year-old took off on her own with her floaties. I actually had a moment to take stock.

I felt my tension reduce. I began to feel some sense of the calmness that comes when you realise that far from being judged, you are being supported: by the pool, the women and the natural beauty of the Baths. I swam out to my daughter who was happily floating, on her own, to the other side of the pool. I smiled and relaxed in the cool, clear water. We spotted a shy crab as it scuttled under some rocks.

As we were leaving, we met their grandmother who was just arriving for a swim. We stayed with her and her group of friends while she changed, quite unselfconsciously, into her red swimsuit. She placed her clothes in a neat bundle and covered them with her towel.

The girls giggled and talked to the other women who seemed to enjoy their playfulness. I looked at these women and realised that they too must have hard things to do at times, probably much harder than taking two girls to a safe place for a swim. I know that children absorb knowledge from their surroundings and the people that they love and I know that I want them to be here often, with these women, in this place.

At home, children safely napping, I thought about this first venture to the pool, where I found acceptance and reassurance. I hoped that it would influence my daughters as it had influenced me. I determined to make time to do some volunteering at the pool — just to contribute in some way. Yes, they start them young there, but you can benefit from being at the women's pool — anytime.

*Joanne Fedler writes of her goal to achieve safety for women and children — and finding its quintessence at the women's pool.*

# Safety: Where the Outside Meets the Inside

## Joanne Fedler

I ARRIVED AS AN IMMIGRANT TO AUSTRALIA in October 2001, weeks after 9/11, with two toddlers and a splintered heart. We left everyone we loved and everything that shaped us in South Africa, after an incident of violence ripped like a chainsaw through my family. For that is what it takes to uproot us — a catastrophic undoing.

We landed at the Medina apartments in Randwick while we waited for our shipment of furniture to arrive. I couldn't believe our luck: Coogee beach was only a short walk down the hill.

One evening, my husband found me ragged with exhaustion and he encouraged me to go out for a walk. I made my way down Alison Road to the beach, where I sat by myself as dusk crept in. I looked out across the ocean and let the sadness and homesickness, which I kept concealed from my kids, rise up in my heart. It was getting dark, but people were out and about. Never before had I been alone on a beach at night. I wondered if I should be scared. Something I didn't recognise sidled up close; it settled around me, an unfamiliar presence. It took me a moment to identify the feeling, like scrambling to remember the name of someone not seen for years. It was *safety*. I lay back in the sand and spread my arms wide to the sky. For this, we'd sacrificed everything to bring our children here. I sobbed with relief.

In South Africa, I'd been an advocate to end violence against women. Somewhere in my late teens, a line from Mary Oliver's poem, *Small Bodies*, imprinted itself in me, "Still there are so many small bodies in the world for which I am afraid." The safety of women and children is what I have cared most about, but it has proved to be the most elusive goal of my life.

I have always tried to imagine what real safety might look and feel like for women in a world of toxic masculinity and emasculated, angry, traumatised people. The secret location of shelters for abused women seemed the closest approximation but, like witness protection programmes, they are fraught with their own problems. It is eviscerating and exhausting to remain in hiding; there is no relief to be found there for the innocent.

I'd experienced women-only spaces in regional meetings of women's organisations that spanned socio-economic, ethnic, and racial lines. We shared ideas, banded together to pressure the government to change laws, and advocated for more resources. Many activists were survivors of sex-based violence; warriors, broken once, but soldered on with grit.

Our gatherings were always political as we debated how to stop rape, domestic violence, sexual assault and femicide. Everything was at stake as we wrestled for equality and our daughters' and sons' futures.

This was long before 2011 when Eve Ensler (now 'V', and author of the *Vagina Monologues*) helped establish the City of Joy in the Democratic Republic of Congo, modelling what a safe haven for women survivors might look like: a whole township dedicated to women's healing. Here women are stitched back together — physically and emotionally — and, through dancing, singing and workshops, they become empowered leaders in their communities. The ten founding principles form a feminist anthem, with number ten declaring: *Treat your sisters' life as if it were your own.* To see every woman as a sister — this, perhaps more than anything, is the essence of what makes a woman feel welcome, safe.

We'd been in Australia for a few years when I heard a confidence — passed from woman to woman, friend to friend — that there was a women-only ocean baths in Coogee. It sounded like a secret club, a cult, for which a special invitation or a password was needed. I don't remember the first time I ventured down the steps of McIver's Ladies Baths (I've never, frankly, identified as a 'lady' and wondered when modern gender theory might catch up with its name and ethos) but it was back when entry involved aiming a 20 cent piece through the bars of the security gate, hoping it would land in the big blue bucket.

As I took in the sight of the secluded pool, tucked in the embrace of the cliff, with girls and women sprawled on the grass and draped on rocks like four-limbed starfish, some topless, some in full coverage burkinis, I exhaled deeply. There were, it appeared, still spaces in the world which were set aside just for us, created by and for women only: zones free from the male gaze; places the Indigenous people of this land reserve for 'secret women's business.'

The felt experience of admission to such locations is visceral, energetic; something *happens* in our bodies. Only when we step through the gates and the gravity of objectification lifts like a leaden x-ray blanket, do our limbs lighten, our torsos untense. Only then does the insidious, invisible stress of what we feminists call 'the patriarchy' drop away.

Since that day, the women's pool has rooted itself as a compass point for my life — not just for my body, but my spirit.

Here is where I held a special ritual for my 12-year-old daughter with a group of women for her *batmitzvah* in 2009. We gathered on the grass and each of us presented her with a gift that cost no money, which embodied what womanhood means to us. Then we fed her fruits she'd never tasted before — longans and custard apple — before we all bounded into the water, strewn with rose petals.

Another year, around Christmas time, I left a box full of copies of my book *When Hungry, Eat* in the changeroom with a note, 'HELP YOURSELF' and smiled when I returned to find them all taken.

I conducted a *mikvah* ritual for a friend to cleanse her of an icky divorce and to ready her for a second marriage. We laid her on a sari, bestowed her with blessings and poems, and celebrated with cake and song.

Each year, on my birthday, the day before spring, I have met with a few friends for a 'birthday dunk.' With the late August water still icy, this invariably involves screeching and shrieking, and the imperative "putting your head under," otherwise it "doesn't count."

Some days though, the ship of my life seemed to be sinking and I felt utterly separate from a sense of home and community. I was marooned from friendship and family. My eyes were blurred from screens; the news was grim. And I'd remember — the Baths. To the Baths.

There I'd loosen my breasts, float free, undo my hair until it was a stream of dark tangles down my back, and I'd cry in the water until I couldn't tell what were tears and what was ocean, and by then, what did it matter?

There, I learned to love my own ageing body more, and to appreciate the muscled, sinewed, wizened, wondrous bodies of all who come here to lay down their sorrows and lift their chins to the sunshine. In every body that comes here to be free, I sense what freedom could be in the world outside its gates.

At the pool, I also learned to love the body of the octopus, curled into the nook of the rock, the exoskeleton of the starfish, the grace of the cormorant — are they our visitors or are we theirs?

In 2018 a back injury left me unable to move for a full seven weeks. When I could finally walk short distances, I made my way to the ocean, for those moments of weightless relief. Since then, I have swum every day, come wind or rain, regardless of the air or water temperature.

I used to avoid the shock of cold water. Now I crave it.

On one occasion, I stood patiently as an elderly woman, ahead of me on the stairs, struggled to get in. "Too cold," she shivered.

"It makes me feel so alive," I replied. "Menopause," I added as I dived in, literally sizzling like a blazing horseshoe dipped in water. "Besides, cold is good — when the ocean heats up, our planet will be in big trouble," I called back to her.

"That's a good way to think of it," she said, as she took the plunge.

One day, I sat at the Baths on the sentry of rocks, writing in my journal, as a young woman in her early 20s squeezed past me to find a spot. She settled on a ledge beneath me, stripped off her bikini top and opened a book. I didn't catch the title but the chapter heading was 'Facing Trauma'. On another outcrop, a young woman with a skin condition that covered her entire body sunned herself in a bikini.

One of the volunteers once remarked that lots of teenage girls are coming to the pool these days — to "get away from the nonsense," as she put it. "Women who've been abused, you know."

"Oh, I know," I nodded.

Until I swam here, I never went nipple-to-water. But here, naked breasts are not performative or a form of exhibitionism. They are a gesture of self-recovery, of self-celebration. Those who have lost their hair from cancer treatment, orthodox Muslim and Jewish women in their long-sleeved full coverage — and those of every age, shape and size — disrobe, splash and stretch themselves out, with a fearlessness that sometimes brings me to tears.

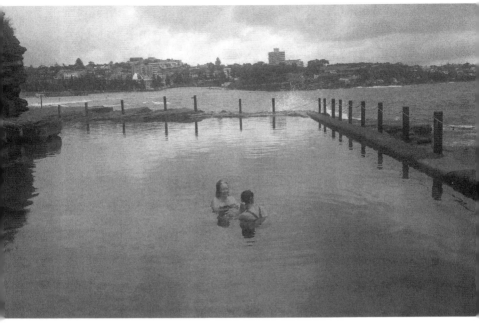

*Sisterhood*
Photograph by Wendy Freeman

Here, we come to feel our life force flow back into us, like a new tide, as we are enfolded in a welcome that is ecological, historical. Here is a sense of a long ancestral heritage, deeper than blood family, broader than just human bodies, an alchemy of rock and wind and water and fish and crustacean and octopodidae and mammal.

It comforts me to know this place has been here for eons before me and will remain long after I am gone. How lucky we are to have inherited this sanctuary, and to pass it on and down to the girls and women who will need it. Heaven, I believe, will be something like this — sloshing, dreamy, salt-winded, light-speckled and enfolding.

This 'holy' spot in Coogee remains an escape from the noise and torments of the world beyond the pool. Here women are mermaided, sistered to one another in safety, until the outside meets us with the freedoms our bodies have come to cherish, on the inside.

*A long recovery from illness — and the Thursday Married Ladies'
Club.*

# Swimming, Cigarettes and Sex

## Wendy Assinder

THE WORLD'S WORST HEADACHE was hammering from
deep within my skull, as if it wanted to explode out between
my eyes. The most poisonous hangover could not compare
with this. Nor did the car accident I'd once endured. This
headache was unrelenting and had been pounding away
almost incessantly for six months. It was one of the many
symptoms of a tick-borne illness I had contracted while
travelling, not in some exotic faraway destination like the
Kalahari Desert or the Amazon rainforest, but in Australia's
Northern Territory.

As I regained consciousness from my opiate-induced
slumber, I became aware of another pounding: the waves
crashing against the rocks. I remembered that I was at
McIver's Baths, just across the road from my rather dark
basement apartment in Beach Street, Coogee — in which I
had spent the last few months confined to my bed, battling
alternate high fevers and bone-rattling attacks of shivering.

In my debilitated state, I had struggled the short distance to the ocean pool so that I could sunbathe for a while on a rock, and inhale some salt air.

The rock was a very large piece of Sydney sandstone, and I was lying nestled into an indentation created by centuries of waves and weathering. I had put my shoes and towel under my head as a makeshift pillow and was positioned with a north-western aspect, so that the early-afternoon sun was on my face. Having spent my youth in England, I was grateful for the warmth. I had recently stumbled upon the word 'Apricate' (*verb: to bask in the sun*), and this is exactly what I was doing: *apricating*. If only the headache would go away. Even for a while. It didn't. I opened my eyes and squinted at the world, which all seemed a bit surreal. Everything was so bright: the azure of the pool water, the silver laminate on the waves, the sparkling mica in the yellow rock, the deep blue Sydney sky, and the colourful swimsuits and caps of the various women swimming and splashing. It was all rather hazy, like a shimmering mirage. I wondered whether I would be able to get home without embarrassing myself by vomiting. I managed it, just, and went back to bed for another week.

Summer progressed, and the headache remained a constant appendage; it was as if my head was bound with a piece of equipment from a Tuscan torture museum. I made a personal goal to get to the pool, and the rock, every couple of days. Sometimes that was my only excursion away from my subterranean bedroom. Being a creature of habit, I always headed for the same spot. If I could reach the hollow in the big rock, I felt I had accomplished something. The curvature of the depression seemed personally sculpted for my body, and the mere action of reclining in it provided some relief, albeit fleeting. Occasionally, someone else would be lying there, and I would be forced to walk further south along the chain of rocks between McIver's and Wylie's Baths, in search of another stony retreat. In time, I knew each boulder; they welcomed me like friends. There were some deep chasms between the outcrops, tricky to negotiate in my unsteady state, and on one traversal I slipped and cut both knees so badly that they took weeks to heal. I almost cried. At least it was a diversion from the headache. Sometimes, I saw water rats. Once, I saw a sea-eagle circling above; it then swooped down almost vertically at incredible speed, picked up a rat and flew off.

This became my routine. Make it to the rock. Lie down for an hour or two. Go back home to bed, totally exhausted. Gradually, I had the odd hour when the headache would lessen. Then the occasional afternoon. But if I over-exerted myself, the throbbing would reappear with a vengeance, and my penance would be bed-ridden internment for more days, or weeks. If it was raining, I had a day off, and rested at home.

With my focus slowly shifting out of my cranial nightmare, I began to notice other people. By late autumn, the tourists had gone, and most of the women I saw were regulars. Faces became familiar. Others were recognisable by their swimsuit or hat, by the colour of their skin or shade of suntan, their tattoos, their gait, or their swimming stroke. Sometimes there was loud banter, and I heard many different accents. I tried not to make eye contact, as I did not have the energy for conversation, but I became aware of varying rhythms of activity: mid-week was very quiet, especially on the rocks; sunny weekends were busier. Often groups of lesbians would traipse down on Saturday and Sunday afternoons, sometimes with six-packs of beer, and sit near me, smoking and chatting. I'd overhear them discussing the 'lezzo' venues of the time (mid-1990s): The Bank Hotel, The Lizard Lounge, The Cricketers Arms, and others. They'd talk about who they'd met, how much they'd drunk and who they'd gone home with. I wondered if I'd ever be well enough to go out to a restaurant or nightclub again, let alone go home with anyone. Another group was clearly some university students majoring in Gender Studies. They'd bring along interesting looking books, and have deep debates. One woman was undergoing gender reassignment, female to male. I thought she was very brave, and wondered how long she, or he, would be able to come to McIver's. (Now, of course, I would say, "I thought *they* were very brave and wondered how long *they* would be able to come here.")

The far end of the tract of rocks was quite sheltered from the main pool area, with some private nooks and crannies between boulders, and occasionally I would witness amorous antics. How refreshing, I thought, to have a women-only space where this could actually happen, in the open air, with a Pacific view. I would close my eyes, and smile.

On Thursdays, I noticed that a large group of mostly older, white Australian women would congregate in the clubhouse and change into brightly coloured floral swimsuits (of 'supportive' design, not skimpy: *Swimsuitus robustus*, I dubbed them; some even had built-in 'skirts').

The ladies then held noisy swimming races, complete with a starting pistol. They were very competitive, even those in their 70s and 80s, and there was always laughter, a range of expletives as the water got colder, and a glowing camaraderie. These women had clearly been coming here for decades. As I passed the clubhouse on my way home, there would be a line of dripping swimwear and towels drying on the fence outside, and cackles from within the room as the ladies tucked into tuna sandwiches and cakes, shared produce from their gardens, and sometimes guzzled Great Western Champagne out of coloured glasses. The scores of the swimming races were chalked up each week on a blackboard. These Aussie elders looked like interesting characters, no doubt with years of stories, and I longed to know more about them and the history of the pool.

The matriarch of this group of Thursday ladies was an elegant woman in her late eighties, slim, suntanned, and with her silver hair tied back. This was Lorna. She was courteous, always had a big smile, and used a lot of very colourful vernacular expressions. She came every day, not just on Thursdays, and did a few laps of the pool in her black swimsuit and red lipstick. Then she would retire to the clubhouse and spend the afternoon smoking, sipping glasses of wine from the fridge, chatting with other swimming club members, or — if she was alone — listening to the radio. One sunny afternoon in winter, when there were not many people around, she saw me struggling up the stairs and asked me in, to have a cup of tea with her. I was honoured: it was the first time I'd been inside this revered, but simple, establishment. While Lorna was topping up the teapot, my eyes skimmed the walls and I noted a cabinet of trophies, plaques listing winners of various swimming tournaments, photos of bygone days at the pool, and other swimming memorabilia. There was a row of pegs from which hung swimsuits, goggles, towels, rubber caps, and bags of soaps and lotions. On the table were a horse-racing guide, a vase of orange and yellow nasturtiums, and a pile of novels. What a wonderful place.

Unfortunately, I was still quite ill. After the tea, I had an attack of 'the shivers'. Lorna kindly lent me her beautiful red cashmere and merino cardigan to wear, and told me to take it home. It smelt of cigarettes and perfume; I wanted to keep it, but of course I returned it the next day. After that, we started having little chats when we crossed paths. She mentioned a friend of hers who had had Ross River fever, with similar symptoms to the ones I had from tick typhus. She told me how she had been born in Broken Hill, far from the ocean, but had come to Sydney 60 odd years ago when she married Bob, who was still alive and who spent his afternoons just down the road at Coogee Surf Club, drinking 'brown lemonade'. She spoke of going to the Melbourne Olympic Games in 1956 as a spectator, and talked about various Coogee characters and McIver's personalities. We became friends.

A couple of years later, I was invited to her ninetieth birthday party. What was the secret to her longevity, she was asked. Her reply came without missing a beat: "Swimming, cigarettes, and sex!", she beamed.

*A regular at the pool, Mary Goslett determines to find out more about the famous Thursday Married Ladies Club.*

# The Thursday Married Ladies' Club

## Mary Goslett

THURSDAY HAS TRADITIONALLY BEEN 'MARRIED LADIES DAY' at the women's pool, and until very recently women gathered in the clubhouse for a shared lunch — whether in the chill of mid-winter or on a day of searing heat. The club seems to have been an institution since the early days of McIver's — and a husband was never actually a membership requirement. In fact, many of the 'married ladies' turned to the club after they had lost a partner. There were, and are, members who experienced world wars, decades of social change, personal joys and tragedies and the slow emancipation of women.

I had heard wonderful stories about the group and I wanted to know more about them, to record their stories. Over time, these women formed the core of the volunteers who cleaned the clubhouse and change-rooms and toilets.

They gardened, swept paths, collected entrance fees, liaised with Randwick Council, and welcomed each day's attendees. They were the heart of the community that grew around the pool.

For years, the Thursday ladies arrived with their lunches and usually something to share, a homemade cake or slice or biscuits, and they would settle around the clubhouse table in a joyful flock. Their chirrup and chatter were a welcome soundtrack for the women coming to the pool. In the club's heyday, before all the stringent rules and regulation, so many women appeared on Thursdays at lunch time that they spilled out onto the small grassed area outside. There is an old and damaged photograph showing 25 women, almost all grey-haired, at one of their Thursday meetings.

They participated in organised swimming races, accompanied by cheers and sometimes jeers. Apparently, there was a woman who determinedly took part in the races but "… could not swim straight and caused chaos." Another woman insisted on swimming back and forth across the pool even though everyone else swam up and down its length. Winners' names were proudly displayed on gilded honour boards and trophies were exhibited around the small clubhouse. As the women got older and their joints stiffer, the races faded away. Competition, however, remained fierce, and the members could get points for simply turning up and for getting in the water.

Membership of the Thursday Married Ladies Club was fluid, but there was a core of long-term stalwarts who formed abiding connections. All the current members are resilient, unpretentious women who have lived long and sometimes difficult lives; all have made the pool part of their existence and contributed to it without question.

They regale each other with stories of past gatherings, of friends who have passed on, parties that were moved into the cavernous change room because there were so many people, and lunches lubricated by wine (in the days before alcohol was prohibited). I sat with two of the 'married ladies' to ask about the club and they agreed that it was about swimming and fun, but mostly about community. They told of morning teas to raise money for charities and of the nuns from Brigidine and Sacred Heart convents who came down to swim, their modesty matched by the Muslim women who also came for privacy.

One told of a day she and a friend arrived early, "worked up a good sweat" as they cleaned the toilets and change rooms and then went down to the pool for a cool-off swim. They were met with the vision of a three-seater lounge in the pool, fully submerged. She rang her son who worked at the local council, and a group of men turned up and, "stripped to their daks, jumped in and grabbed the lounge and manhandled it out of the pool and up the stairs." They never discovered how the lounge got there. She then told of the time when dog-poo bags were first introduced to Coogee. She and her friend arrived to do the cleaning. As always, once finished, they dived in for their much anticipated cool-off, to find the bottom of the pool littered with black plastic dog-poo bags — complete with contents. And the poo-bag stand had also been thrown in. As they talked of the toil of removing the muck, they asked what would make someone do this. They told of the darker history of the pool:

the graffiti, the smeared faeces on the walls and the several times in the 1970s when the clubhouse was deliberately set on fire. It seems that some people simply cannot accept that women should legally have something to themselves.

One of these women is now 84 years old. She doesn't swim very often because of the steep stairs to the pool but she still attends the Thursday Club. She was from England and met her husband when they were both working on cruise ships. He was from Coogee and at the age of 30 she came to Australia to be with him. They lived in Lithgow for a while, where her sons learned to swim in the indoor pool. When they moved back to Coogee, her youngest son still wouldn't put his face under water and someone suggested she take him to the women's pool. After just two lessons with the experienced women teachers, he was able to swim fully submerged.

She says she loved the pool and the opportunity it gave her to meet new people. She joined in the freestyle races even though she only knew breaststroke and, laughingly, tells of finally winning a trophy because she had the most points accumulated for 'participation'.

This woman talks with regret of the changes that have occurred at the pool. So many people, so many rules and regulations: "It's too regimented." She lists the names of women who have gone, particularly the kind ones who took time to offer cups of tea and a quiet talk to those who looked lost. They were part of the old-school brigade who gave freely of their time, energy, cheer and warmth.

The second 'married lady' is 79. She has unlocked the pool buildings nearly every morning since the 1970s and has been a mainstay of the Thursday Club — as it has been for her through hard times. Until recently, the outside pool gate was not locked overnight, and women could access the pool at all hours. Sometimes there were overnight interlopers who took advantage: lounge throwers, aspiring graffiti artists and occasional vandals. But the unlocked gate ensured the women's place was there when its comfort and peace were needed. You would be surprised, the married ladies told me, at the number of women who relished the opportunity for a night swim, especially by moonlight.

For 50 years, this early-bird arrived before sunrise and made her way down in the dark to unlock the doors to the clubhouse and the change room. If they needed cleaning (and they often did), she would clean them. Then, the reward: the dawn swim. Whatever the temperature, she'd swim her laps, savouring the solitary pleasure of a pool to herself; so cold in winter's 'night-water' but silk-like when the tide comes in, bringing warm water.

The Thursday Married Ladies Club still meets, although changes to pool management rules and the limitations imposed by COVID have sent them at lunch-time on Thursdays to the park opposite Coogee beach. If you want to know more about the history of McIver's and the lives of the women who have maintained the pool as a welcoming and nurturing place, you can find them there, after their swim in the Ross Jones (mixed bathing and male-named) pool, sitting around a table, under a shelter. You'll recognise them because they will be sharing lots of food and will probably be laughing. I have never asked them what is in their stylish, non-see-through water bottles.

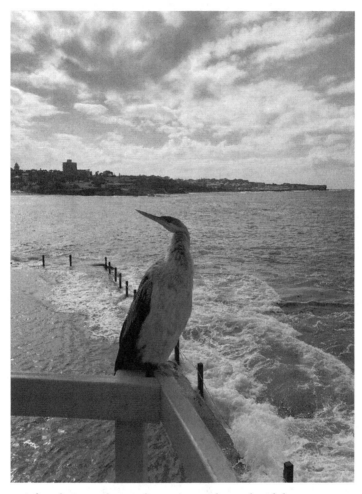

*A female Australasian darter graces the pool with her presence*
Photograph by Wendy Assinder

*Raised in an institution as a 'home' kid, Colleen found her first warmth and kindness at the Thursday Married Ladies Club.*

# Mrs C and the Thursday Married Ladies' Club

## Colleen Kelly

MRS C GENTLY SLIDES THE PLATE TOWARDS ME with a, "Here you go darlin', help us finish this cake off, will ya? Look at you — all skin and bone. Don't they feed you in that place?" Some 60 years later, I'm sitting in that same room at another Thursday Married Ladies Club lunch, and cake is still gently being pushed towards me with a soft "Finish this cake off, will you, it's not worth taking home."

From my first bite of cake all those years ago, women and food have been at the very heart of my relationship with McIver's Ladies Baths, its women, its circle of giving and my life experiences.

Let's take a moment to start at the beginning. At the age of 12, I started at Randwick Public School in Avoca Street. I hated school — not just Randwick, but all schools. I couldn't read or write, I was always in the remedial class (the bottom) and felt like an outsider. I was committed to spending as little time as possible within any school walls, so I used to wag school and go surfing.

I would walk to school from Paddington, spending my bus fare on a warm, white bread bun from the bakery across the road in Avoca Street. Once all the other pupils had filed in, I would head down Frenchman's Road to Coogee beach. There I would hide under the boats on the northern end where I kept my stash (surfboard, tobacco etc), and wait until most of the people had gone. Then I would either surf, wander around, talk to other kids or go up the hill to the Ladies Baths, which I had found by accident one day while walking aimlessly. Luckily for me, that day happened to be a Thursday, when the ladies sat around eating, drinking tea, chatting and laughing.

I soon learnt, however, that Thursday was *the* day to drop in, because Mrs C was there. I liked Mrs C. She was a short old lady with white curly hair, who would look kindly at me when she spoke to me. Mrs C would always find a chair or make room for me near her. She would rub my back softly and slowly as she laughed and chatted with her lady friends. When I was cold, she would wrap me in a towel and rub me hard and fast until I got warm. Then she would give me cake. Before Mrs C, I had never experienced softness, and after a day of cake and Mrs C, I always left feeling taller and tingling all over. She was nice to me, and I loved it.

You see, the home I grew up in was an institution. These 'homes' for children were mostly run by the government but sometimes a 'well meaning' private citizen would start one. The one I was in was run by one man, and there were 84 of us kids. I was the youngest. It was tough and brutal; there was absolutely no room, time or capacity for softness, or even fairness. In those days, no one liked 'home' kids. People said if a kid is in a home, they must have done something to deserve it; there must be something bad about them if even their mother doesn't want them. As a result, I grew up an outsider.

So, Mrs C giving me cake and being nice to me was exceptional. My first humane experience. I know it was big because 60 years later I still see and feel Mrs C every time I walk into McIver's Baths.

My long-ago Thursday visits went on for about a year until I was expelled from the school at Randwick and was moved overnight to one of the other 'homes' in Manly. I lost Mrs C. Just like that. I never saw her again.

I hated Manly; it was hard and lonely. For years, when things were really bad, I would sneak down to the water and imagine Mrs C rubbing my back to keep me warm and giving me cake to feel better. She had never once failed to comfort me. You see, when I lost Mrs C and the Ladies Baths, I lost the only physically and emotionally safe space I had ever known. For years I ached for Thursdays with Mrs C and the other ladies; and yes, if I'm honest, I missed the cake.

Over the past 60 years, the spirit of Mrs C has kept me company, not as a guest or passenger, but as a fellow traveller. She has always been there in the background guiding, comforting and providing me with an example of relating to others that I still use today. There have been many times when I stopped what I was about to do and asked myself, "Would Mrs C be happy with you doing that?"

As the years passed, I became determined to honour and acknowledge Mrs C's kindness in some way. I wanted to complete the circle of giving, commenced by Mrs C and those Thursday ladies over 60 years ago; to give back to the women's pool community that had given so much to me as a very troubled 13-year-old.

After my retirement, I moved to the South Coast, and Mrs C is still with me there today. One day, though, I decided I had to fulfil my promise and I drove to Coogee and presented myself at the Baths and asked how could I contribute to its community.

My giving back to the Baths has centred on three main areas: utilising my building skills as a 'fix-it' person attending to minor repairs, volunteering for general duties, and as a member of the Thursday Married Ladies Club. I have loved and cherished all three roles, however, my time eating Mrs C's cake on Thursdays and recently, as an invited member of the Thursday Married Ladies Club, are the stand-outs.

Sadly, in the past 12 months my relationship with the Baths has dramatically altered. It has changed to a point where I no longer want to be there, because it hurts too much. Some of those overseeing the Baths seem to have lost sight of its value as an envelope of safety for those who need to be part of a real community.

I don't feel safe there anymore and I'm angry. I'm angry because I know my Mrs C would be so sad at this change to her beloved Baths, and she would want it to return to the simple, welcoming place of belonging that it once was. She would certainly scoff at the 50+ signs that are displayed — plastered, more like it — over the walls. As though safety depended on signs and regulations rather than women working collaboratively and as a community.

For some time, I was numb and lost and didn't fully understand why — and I didn't know what to do with this loss and anger. However, in the past six months I've been part of a small group of gentle, caring and strong women from the Baths, fighting hard to 'get our pool back'. Back into the welcoming arms of the many women who have become separated from its embrace.

Our struggle to get our pool back, has been at times exhausting, often maddening, but behind every late night, or frustrating discussion, has been Mrs C's gentle guiding hand. Although I never actually knew her name — I called her 'Mrs Cake' in my head, shortened to Mrs C — I know without a doubt, there have been several times in my life when, without her spirit to comfort and guide me, my life would have been lost.

It has taken the near loss of our beloved Baths community for me to fully comprehend just how important my time, although brief, with Mrs C and the Thursday Married Ladies has been in my life and I'm sure the same is true for countless of other women. It is this understanding and appreciation that drives my determination to continue the fight for our pool so that the circle of women caring for women, started all those years ago, can continue.

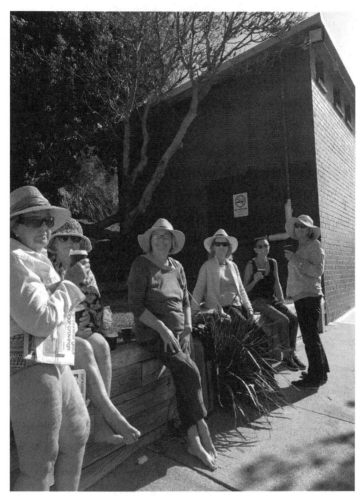

*Some of the regulars*
Photograph by Sheila Abrahams

*For decades before the employment of 'ocean baths attendants' and before TripAdvisor promoted the women's pool as a tourist destination, volunteer 'guardians' managed the women's pool; opening and closing, cleaning, caring for the bushland, supporting other women who came to the pool for safety, privacy and pleasure. They were assisted for a few seasons by summer coordinators who left their own mark on the pool community.*

# Scenes from the Women's Pool

## Lynne Spender

### THE SUMMER COORDINATORS

### I

### *On duty*

A FLASH OF RED AND PURPLE. A woman in a hurry.

Dark-haired, slight, the morning Coordinator hastens down the stairs of the pool to the locked grille of the clubhouse. She checks inside, then moves to the grassy area outside the change room where she has the best view of the pool. She stops, places her hands on the rails and breathes in sensually as she surveys the pool and the ocean vista. She's a successful artist in her other life and catalogues details that others simply don't see. Below, a gentle ocean swell sends water rippling over the rocks, outside the pool. Lots of people and a gentle buzz of activity rises from below. Medium tide offers safe swimming. Quite a few people in the water or sitting on the outside wall of the pool. No loud music or voices. No queues at the toilet. Good.

She heads back to the clubhouse and slips inside, dumps her shoulder bag on the table and pulls out a bright yellow singlet labelled 'Pool Coordinator'. She hauls her peacock shirt over her head and pulls on the singlet. Runs her hand through her curly hair and checks the money in the blue bin which sits within throwing distance of the locked grille door. Swimmers who arrive before the Coordinator are asked, via a large sign, to throw their $2 into the bin. Most do but some look around stealthily and pass by without paying.

As well as the coins that have made it into the bin, there are many on the floor. It's obvious the throwers are swimmers and not basketballers. She checks the people counter on the wall. Ninety comings and goings already registered since the early morning opener reset it. She scoops up the coins from the bin with a child's plastic spade and tips them into the metal safe, spilling some on the floor. Damn. She picks them all up and there's a call from the doorway. One of the trained volunteers has arrived. The Coordinator grins. "Hiya. Come on in." She has an untrained newbie coming today as well. It's going to be busy. And the tide is coming in.

The volunteer knows what to do. She tucks her own bag into the corner of the clubhouse and picks up a plastic container, taped around with bright yellow tape. She changes her own t-shirt for a yellow 'Volunteer' shirt and hauls a plastic chair outside. She greets some new arrivals, holding out the yellow container for their coins. They move on, eager to find a spot to settle. A woman with two small children arrives; it looks like she's coming to stay overnight. As well as a stroller and a fold-up chair, she has towels, blankets, an esky, hats and bags. She can't find her purse in all the paraphernalia. More people start to queue behind her. The volunteer explains that the pool will put in $2 for her from the 'pay-forward' jar and she can pay and replace the donated $2 next time. In the next tranche of arrivals, someone has a $50 note and the Coordinator miraculously comes up with the 'float' and provides the right amount of change. The caravan moves on.

Inside the clubhouse, the Coordinator signs in and puts her lunch box in the fridge. Looks inside the fridge. *Ugh*. It needs cleaning. Maybe later. She turns back to her bag of surprises and pulls out a container of home-made cookies (her own) and a jar of jellybeans. She likes to have treats to offer during the day. It's welcoming. Like the fabled cottage in the wood. There's even a resident fox. She's seen it several times and always feels a sort of empathy with the fox as it boldly meets her gaze and then slinks off.

The new volunteer recruit arrives on time. The Coordinator knows not to rush her with information and instructions. Better to just show her around and talk quietly about the tasks she will be asked to carry out over the next few hours.

The tasks aren't onerous but when the pool reaches capacity — and it could today, judging by the weather forecast of 30 degrees — tensions sometimes arise. And smokers. The Coordinator has a 'thing' about smokers. There are several signs saying NO SMOKING, but some will try it on anyway. They drive her crazy. Even though she's been to a de-escalation workshop and knows (in theory) not to confront in anger, she has to bite her lip and count to ten when she sees them smoking and flicking their cigarette butts onto the rocks or into the bushland around the pool. Some are defiant and she is aware of an almost uncontrollable urge to pluck the cigarettes from their mouths. Of course, she resists.

She guides the new recruit around the pool grounds, making her way between the already sun-exposed bodies. She speaks to a group who are spreading their bags and towels across the path and asks that they move them, to allow people to move through safely. The pathways are far from pristine. There's already been one swimmer this year who broke an ankle when her foot slipped off the path. The local council does maintenance but the paths are uneven on the steep ground.

The new recruit follows dutifully along a path that leads to steps up to the private sunbathing area where there are huge NO SMOKING signs on the bare concrete walls. A request to paint a mural on the walls, maybe an Indigenous work to celebrate the original users of the pool, was rejected on the grounds that it might encourage graffiti. She explains quietly to the recruit that it's a good idea to include this area when doing the rounds. Sometimes there are disagreements about space and noise and, in spite of the signs, it is not uncommon for someone to light up.

There are several women lying quietly, soaking up the sun. Some of them wear G-strings. She nods to those who look up. She would like to check whether they have sunscreen on but hey, they are grown-ups. Her job does not include advice on avoiding skin cancer.

They retreat from the sun trap, through some carefully tended native bushes, down another set of stairs, to the point where the pool meets the rugged and ragged rock formation to the south. A wit has described this summer spectacle as the 'seal colony'. It's an apt description. Already there is bevy of tanned and oiled creatures lying, sitting, sleeping, wriggling to find a comfortable place. A rookery. There is a particular smell that accompanies their suntan lotion. Not unpleasant, but it overwhelms the scent of sea spray and native shrubs. The Coordinator knows that later she will have to scoop the coagulated remains of oleaginous sunscreen lotion from the corner of the pool. The tide will deal with the oil slick on the surface. She calls to a group of women making their way across the rocks. "Take care. It can be dangerous!"

She leads the newbie down a further set of irregular steps and the pool comes into full view. It never ceases to amaze her how beautiful it is, even when being lashed by huge swells and high tides. There's something primal about it. Today it is benign and the ocean beyond has a Mediterranean look. No problems here. There are too many people in the water for anyone to actually swim laps, as the early morning regulars do. Less confident and older bathers bob up and down in the shallower parts of the pool. The self-assured swimmers call them 'the teabags'.

The Coordinator notes that a few young women have their phones with them, taking selfies. There is a No Photography rule at the pool. It's impossible to enforce these days, with almost everyone carrying a smart phone. She muses that the idea of privacy has changed. Mobile phones. Selfies. She tells the new volunteer that she doesn't interfere if swimmers are just taking photos of each other. Who wouldn't want to record their experience at the pool?

She thinks ahead and realises that on the way back to the clubhouse, she should go to the large change room and check the toilet and the sanitary bin. Replacing the toilet paper will be good training for the recruit. Someone has left their swimmers hanging from a peg in one of the shabby shower cubicles so she collects them to take to lost property. She could probably start a swimming costume stall at the markets. She explains the lost property protocol to the new volunteer then suggests a quick but reassuring cup of tea and some cookies. It's important to keep the volunteers happy and positive.

Back at the clubhouse the Coordinator checks that the volunteer on duty is managing the increasing number of women lining up to enter the pool. The volunteer is dealing with a woman who wants her 14-year-old nephew to be allowed in. He's just turned 14. The woman decries the 'stupid rule' that says boys over 13 are not permitted. The woman threatens to complain to the Randwick Council. The volunteer says that she thinks it's a good idea. The woman and the boy turn and go back up the stairs.

The Coordinator wonders if she will have to put the POOL CLOSED sign up today. There is a limit to the number who can safely be accommodated. There is a disturbance at the door. A young woman has fallen on the rocks and scraped her shin and wrist. Lots of blood. She makes a quick assessment and sees that it looks worse than it is but there is a kerfuffle as the woman and her friends crowd into the clubhouse. The Coordinator firmly points out that she will need some space to administer first aid, and they retreat, causing confusion with the new arrivals who are jostling to get past to find a spot in the sun. She catches the eye of the volunteer on duty at the entrance and raises an eyebrow. The volunteer gives her the thumbs up. She's an old hand and manages to sort it out quickly and without fuss. The Coordinator turns back to the patient and, while she cleans and applies antibiotic ointment to the scrapes, she light-heartedly tells of her escapade the night before with a new man. She leaves the new recruit to apply bandaids and looks at the clock. It's 10.50. Still a long way to go.

## II

## *The best job ever*

A CLATTER AND "SORRY, SORRY, CAN I GET THROUGH?" A tall suntanned woman, young, with long dark hair tied up in a knot, makes her way down the stairs with a bicycle. There are a few women on the stairs and they step aside to let her through. The volunteer on duty gives her an awkward hug, bicycle between them. They laugh.

She manoeuvres the bike through the clubhouse door and places it against the far wall as much out of the way as possible. She'd leave her bike up the top, but she's already had one stolen. Not here at the pool. But as she says, "Once bitten …"

The morning Coordinator quickly provides a summary of events. No real trouble. The pool is close to capacity. Most of the regulars have departed and the remaining hordes are packed in tightly. Always a recipe for possible trouble. She can't help exploding about a group who have been smoking and who have been difficult when challenged. "Watch out for them. They're just on the rocks at the south end. Young and mouthy," she says. "Oh — and someone in the sunbathing area has a boombox. They turn it down when I appear but then turn it up again. Just keep an eye out?"

The new Coordinator puts on her yellow t-shirt revealing long and strong arms. She's not a native beach girl but feels a complete affinity with the pool and its surrounds. She's swum at Hampstead Ladies' Pond in London and knows the joy of a women's pool. She's been swimming here at McIver's since she came to Australia and was eager to get this job when it was advertised. Even if she does have to ride ten kilometres to get here. It's close to her idea of heaven. Except when it's not. It takes quite a bit to get her riled or discombobulated but she's been tried a few times.

She can't count the number of times she's had to deal with complaints that a man was sitting on the rocks, watching the pool and the women sunbathing. At times, she's confronted a man and found that he was completely unaware that this is forbidden territory. Such men usually go quietly. Others resist and she has to stand to her full height and insist that they leave or she will call the Ranger. Some of them leave. Others argue and even shout abuse. She doesn't back off and mostly, the women around move in to support her. So far, she's prevailed, even when she has felt physically threatened. She's aware that one day it might become ugly. It's an adrenaline trip.

She recalls raising the issue of men in the bushes with binoculars or men exposing themselves to the women on the rocks. Should she call the Police? The Council Rangers?

The regulars didn't take it too seriously. "Been happening forever, darling. He'll be gone by the time the police arrive. Take your camera and pretend to photograph him. He'll go quick smart." She had wanted to say — "but they shouldn't be able to get away with it. It should be stopped." But she realises that the regulars are probably right and the risk comes with the female territory. Not just at the pool. #MeToo.

Looking back on her time as one of the first paid Coordinators at the pool she says there were occasions when she had to assume a disapproving face when someone refused to pay the entry fee (because they 'already pay rates') or someone argued about bringing in their teenage sons. But they were minor perturbations. It was, without doubt, the best job she had ever had. And not just for the pleasure of working outdoors at a place of natural beauty.

She talks wistfully about what she learned about women — and about life. She was amazed at how 'earthy' the older women volunteers were. Unlike the women at home, in England, who would never have felt comfortable talking openly about their lives: about bodies and sex, about their breast cancer and mastectomies; their joys and disappointments. She thinks perhaps it is about the freedom in a women only space to simply be yourself, without artifice and without worrying if you are conforming to the accepted norms of polite female behaviour. And of course, there are the bodies. So many — and so many differences, unselfconsciously revealed. "It's just not like that where I come from. It's so relaxed here and *so* reassuring."

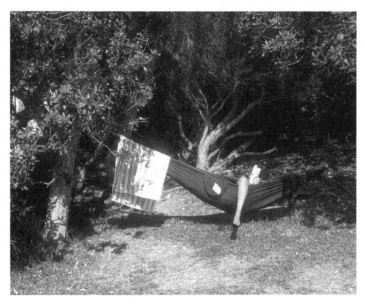

*Relaxing*
Photograph by Wendy Freeman

# THE GUARDIANS

## I

## *The rhythm of life*

SHOULD YOU HAPPEN TO BE at Coogee beach very early in the morning, you will see the stalwarts preparing for their regular swim. Hardy. Tanned. Fit-looking.

Further south, you may glimpse a woman, older, make her way soundlessly through a park to a high green gate. A modest sign says McIver's Baths LADIES AND CHILDREN ONLY. Underneath, a smaller sign: McIver's Ladies Pool. Then: $2 ENTRY, followed by a warning in Capital letters: CHILDREN MUST BE WITH AN ADULT AT ALL TIMES.

Our woman unlocks an old-fashioned padlock and quietly eases open the high green gate. It's still dark and she makes her way carefully down about a dozen steps to the door of the nondescript brick building on her right. More signs. Rules and warnings — NO LIFEGUARDS SWIM AT YOUR OWN RISK. She no longer notices them. She unlocks a grille door and then the locked entry door. She disappears into the dark and switches on the light, revealing the interior of what could be an old but neat and well-kept cottage. She signs her name in an exercise book then reads and writes down the figure on the not very reliable people counter that registers the number of women who enter and leave the pool each day. She fiddles with the counter and resets it.

She emerges from the clubhouse and makes her way along the walkway to the large change room. Again, she unlocks a grille door and an entry door. She checks that all is clean and in order and then shatters the quiet as she unbolts and lifts the roller-door window that looks out over the pool and the ocean. The 'million-dollar view', it's called. She smiles and returns to the clubhouse. There is a noise; a scraping sound as she drags the heavy sandwich board from the clubhouse to the landing outside the door. In bold letters it says '*$2 ENTRY Throw in BIG blue tub in Pool Office*'.

As the darkness recedes and sunlight touches the clubhouse wall, she emerges silently, with towel and bathing cap and closes the grille door and locks it. She makes her way down three sets of irregular steps. She is conscious of falling. If she is lucky she may fleetingly catch sight of the resident fox. She will certainly meet lizards and baby wrens who revel in the native vegetation, so carefully tended by the pool's bush care group.

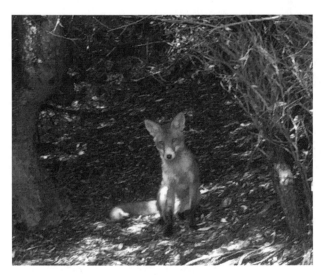

*Resident fox*
Photograph by Wendy Assinder

If you listen, you will hear a gentle splash as she enters the pool. Sometimes the ocean water spills over the north eastern side of the pool. Except in high summer, the sea water is warmer than the pool water. At high tide or when the swell is large, the water pummels over, sweeping towards the rock face from which the pool has been carved. Then she has to be careful, but she knows the pool and its moods. She swims her laps, slowly and methodically. She may perhaps stop to watch the resident octopus lazily extend its tentacles from beneath its rock. After her swim she meets long term friends for a walk, returns to the pool and sits in a comfy chair within sight of the entry. Other morning swimmers arrive and greet her and ask about the water and the tides. She responds, always with a smile, and returns to her book. This is the beginning of her day. It is the rhythm of her life and now, after decades, that of the pool.

## II

### *What's in the tea they are drinking?*

BY THE TIME THE SUN is up, one of the trusted key-holders arrives at the pool. Descending from an eyrie high above the women's pool, she has been to the local café where they know her by name and greet her with an intimacy reserved for special customers. They don't need to ask for her order. She laughingly tells of some overseas mail sent to her 'C/- The café, The Beach, Coogee, Australia'. Of course, they kept it for her. Even the postman knew who she was.

She leaves the café and heads for the pool. She is slight and although her bag looks heavy, she moves easily as she descends the familiar stairs. If no one is yet on duty, she unlocks the grille of the clubhouse and checks inside that all is well. When entry to the pool was still an honour system and women were asked to throw their coins into a bin inside the grille, she was often first to scoop up the coins and place them in the old-fashioned safe — and to collect it all at the end of the day for deposit at the bank. She takes her neatly stored folding chair and relocks the grille. She carries the chair and her bag with her thermos of tea and whale-watching binoculars to her usual spot outside the small wooden changerooms. She unfolds the chair and carefully places her bag beside it. She pulls out a blue thermometer and goes down the uneven stairs to the southern end of the pool to check the water temperature. She collects her blue board-marker, neatly tucked into the side of her bag, and writes the result on the small noticeboard outside the main changeroom. She often adds a message. *Water temperature: 16 degrees: 9 in Tasmania!* She has a sense of humour.

She returns to 'her' spot, protected from the wind. There is a well-worn recess in the grass where she has placed her feet for years. On days when a cold wind is blowing, she miraculously produces a hot-water bottle from her bag and tucks it under her jacket. If or when it becomes warmer, she undresses and heads down for a swim.

Later in the morning as she reads, sips her thermos-tea and triumphantly completes the crossword, she is joined by more women. A magnet. They are the regulars, who volunteer to do the cleaning and the bush care. They sit while they can, sharing tea, food and stories before they swim and head off to their other lives. If someone spots a whale

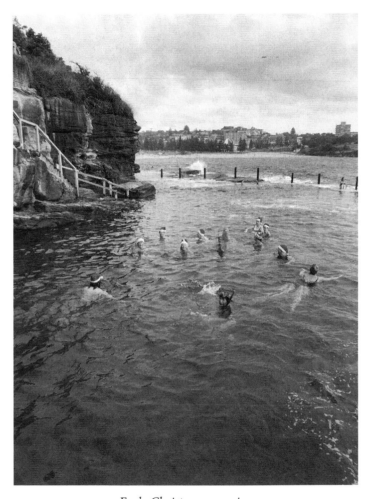

*Early Christmas morning*
Photograph by Wendy Assinder

migrating north to warmer water, there is a frisson of delight as they watch it heave itself out of the water. Binoculars are pulled from the magic bag and confirm *infraorder Cetacea*, probably a humpback. They settle back into an agreeable silence. There is often an outbreak of laughter or a quiet mention of a pool-goer who could do with some help or support. There are sighs of despair about climate change and a recalcitrant government. What will happen to the pool when the sea level rises?

New arrivals with towels and bags walk past the group and look up. They receive welcoming smiles. Many assume the familiar 'lady' in the folding chair is the pool manager, perhaps even the owner, and they often ask her about pool rules and conditions. Mostly, they say shy hellos and wonder who these women are and why they are so often laughing. Younger ones, yet to understand the alchemy of the women's pool, even speculate about what is in the 'tea' that these older women are drinking.

### III

### *Eternal vigilance*

SHE'S TINY — but her size belies her fierce and often outspoken passion for the pool.

The connection to the pool goes way back. For her it's much more than a beautiful and historic place. It's a women's space and its sanctity and principles must be guarded. For all women, always. Eternal vigilance is required.

Mid-morning, she arrives quietly with her sunhat almost eclipsing her face. She has fair skin and is careful to cover up. Not flamboyantly like some of the older women who disport their colourful attire. They say that at their age, it's the only way to be noticed, to make sure they are not 'walked over', physically or metaphorically. It's no surprise that many women come to the pool to avoid the thrashing arms and legs of men who take up so much space in pools and even in the ocean. Beware of aquatic manspreading.

She is transformed when she swims. On calm water days, she slips over the side of the pool with her snorkel and explores the adjacent reef. It may not be elegant to scramble over the rocks and out into the ocean but it's worth the effort. The mini-reef is home to several fabled and protected blue gropers. And schools of 'old wives' — tiny dark brown and white striped fish. The Australian Museum explains that they get their 'derogatory' name from the sound made by grinding their teeth when caught on a hook and line. The name says a lot, she thinks. If she's lucky she'll catch sight of an elusive red fish, plenty of garfish. And stingrays, from babies to the larger more threatening-looking adults, as they glide along the bottom. And of course, there's an occasional hook-up with a grey nurse shark that has given many swimmers a scare. You can pick the swimmers who have seen a grey nurse. They scramble back over the rocks in a hurry.

If you don't know her, it can be a surprise when she speaks out. She has firm ideas on community, equality and women's strength and resilience, ideas crystallised during her time at Amazon Acres, a women only community in northern New South Wales. She has fought ardently for years for the McIver's Ladies Baths to be so much more than just a swimming place for women. It must be a safe place where all are equal and treated with respect. She can be feisty.

She has been an integral part of the evolution of the pool. A quiet activist. Not so long ago, it was a swimming club where a few committed women held swimming classes for children and held exclusive court in the clubhouse. Now it's a fully-fledged incorporated association, obliged to conform to state and local council rules: insurance policies, qualified employees, locked gates and restricted opening times. From relative obscurity to Instagram and TripAdvisor. Not a few of the older women, herself included, sometimes wish it had stayed relatively unknown.

She's a networker who knows most of the women who come regularly and she makes an effort to be kind and welcoming to newcomers. All sorts come to the pool, young and old. It was once a haven for the Randwick nuns who could discard their habits (both literal and traditional) to swim in privacy. And now there are the Muslim women who joyously meet and swim without worrying about being watched or judged. They almost always bring food to share. And take lots of selfies.

She's had occasional altercations with management when they have focused on seemingly arbitrary rules rather than the needs of women. As a firm believer in community and collaboration, it does not sit easily with her when decisions are made at the top without consultation and consensus. Trickle-down management. As damaging as trickle-down economics. She wants to ensure that it's always women's interests that are being served at the glorious women's pool.

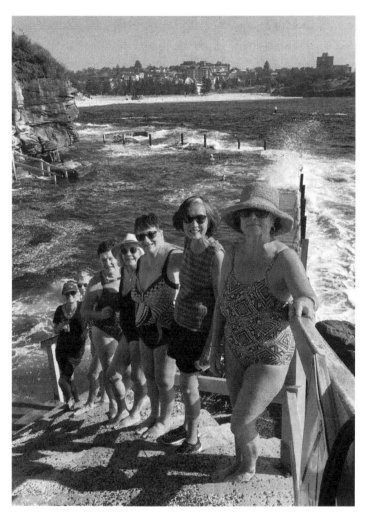

*Guardians of the Pool*
Photograph by Clarissa de Castro Lima

# Biographies

**Wendy Assinder** moved to Coogee from Tokyo in 1988. The upside of many years of poor health is that she has been able to spend extended times convalescing at the McIver's women's pool. She was a member of the Randwick and Coogee Ladies Swimming Club Committee for thirteen years, and is a Life Member of the Association.

**Judy Banki**, is a life-long New Yorker and is an annual visitor to her Aussie family: daughter Susan, a lecturer at the University of Sydney, son-in-law Josh, and two delicious grandchildren. She has spent over half a century working to advance interreligious and intercultural understanding, and to combat religious bigotry. Over the years, she has written and lectured widely in her field, earning many awards and an honorary doctorate. She is an enthusiastic fan of the Ladies Pool, despite being stung by a bluebottle in her first year's visit.

**Susan Banki** is a native New Yorker but has lived near the ocean in Coogee for more than ten years. The ocean is her salve: in her calmest moments she is near the ocean, or in it. She was married at the ocean. And when she dies, hopefully many years in the future, her ashes will be scattered over the ocean.

**Grace Barnes** is a playwright whose work is well known in Scotland where her plays have been produced by the Traverse Theatre Company and The Royal Lyceum in Edinburgh, the Citizens Theatre, Glasgow and Pitlochry Festival Theatre. Grace has written the script for two musicals which have premiered at Signature Theatre, Arlington, USA. She has acted as resident director on large scale musicals in the UK and Australia, and her book on women and musical theatre, *Her Turn on Stage* is published in the US by McFarland Books. In 2018, Grace received her PhD, 'In Search of Mina Wylie', from the University of Technology Sydney.

**Belinda Buchan** is a Coogee swimmer, a teacher and a mother of two daughters. She is a nature-lover and pot-plant wizard and wants her girls to grow into strong, empowered women.

**Josi Crow** is a writer, loudmouth and itinerant fruit picker, bookshop sales assistant, barista, and university student. She hails from Melbourne, currently lives in Sydney and is keen to return to Berlin.

**Tess Durack** is a Sydney-based writer who loves the ocean and the outback in equal measure. After working in the arts for years, she opened a boutique in Darwin before returning to her old neighbourhood of Sydney's eastern 'burbs with her son and setting up shop as a freelance writer. North Bondi is her local stomping (and swimming) ground but you're just as likely to find her roaming the Kimberleys.

**Rhonda Fadden** has lived in Coogee for 30 years — swimming, snorkelling and even diving along the coasts of northern and southern Sydney and in harbour bays. She learned to swim in the creeks around Brisbane and during holidays on the Gold Coast, where there is water, sand and surf, but very few rocky sea pools and no women's pool. She thinks we are very lucky. Rhonda is a member of the Randwick and Coogee Ladies Swimming Association and has volunteered at the Pool.

**Joanne Fedler** is an internationally bestselling author of 13 books which have sold over 750,000 copies worldwide. She is a women's rights activist and writing mentor. Her book *Things Without A Name* (2008) has recently been optioned for a TV mini-series. She lives in Coogee and swims in the ocean every day. <www.joannefedler.com>

**Mary Goslett** is a Yuin Budawang woman who moved to Coogee from the Blue Mountains five years ago. Her moving back to saltwater country was a plan that took many years to achieve, and it was the women's pool that sang to her. She quickly found the community of amazing women at the pool. Mary has a psychology and consultancy practice in Bondi Junction, and plans never to leave the ocean again.

**Colleen Kelly** describes herself as *Myuna Lowanna* (water woman). She lives on the south coast and regularly travels to Sydney to spend time with her pool community.

**Deborah Kneeshaw** says it was love at first sight when she discovered the women's pool twenty years ago. She had relocated to Sydney after a successful career in London as a designer. Her focus here has been on design thinking, working as a trainer and business consultant. You can catch her at the pool most mornings, doing a few of her favourite things: swimming, stretching, chatting with friends and being energised by the ocean. Her other loves include snorkelling, bushwalking and painting.

**Jane Messer** is a writer of fiction and nonfiction. She has published novels, anthologies of world literature and Australian writing; written and produced two radio dramas; and published experimental and realist short fictions including an interactive video game. Her novels *Night by Night*, *Provenance* and *Hopscotch* and radio play *Dear Dr Chekhov* have been critically acclaimed and nominated for national and international awards. She was the Course Director of the Master of Creative Writing at Macquarie University. She is an Honorary Associate Professor in the Department of Media, Communication, Creative Arts, Language and Literature at Macquarie University. She lives in Sydney with her husband and two greyhounds.

**Yusra Metwally** is a community lawyer and writer with a strong policy background. She is passionate about designing programs and policies that achieve social impact.

**Lai Nguyen** was born in Vietnam, but has spent more than half her life in Sydney. She is a keen gardener, and loves cooking spicy food for family, friends and other hungry people. Now retired, she studies English whenever possible, and also enjoys volunteering at McIver's and in community groups such as Bushcare.

**Dominique Pile** is a documentary researcher who would love to be reincarnated as a water sprite. After spending 17 years in Paris and London, she returned to her native Sydney where she discovered love and the Coogee women's pool in close proximity. Both still make her feel alive.

**Helen Pringle** lives in Coogee, and works in the Faculty of Arts and Social Sciences at the University of New South Wales, up the road from McIver's. She often lazes on the rocks at McIver's rather than strenuously swimming. She writes on popular and academic forums about women's rights, sexual violence, freedom of speech, and ethics in public life.

**Maddy Proud** is a professional netballer, currently captaining the NSW Swifts in the Suncorp Super Netball Competition. Maddy has played professionally since the age of 16, the youngest player to be contracted to a professional netball team in the Trans-Tasman ANZ Championships. She is a current member of the Australian Netball Diamonds squad. Her first children's novel, *Grace on the Court,* was published in January 2018 by Piccolo Nero. Maddy has recently completed a Master of Creative Writing at Macquarie University. The sequel to her first novel will hopefully be released in 2021.

**Lynne Spender** is a feminist, a writer and editor, who has lived in and around Coogee for 40 years. She has been a volunteer at the pool, swims all year round and values the pool enough to have undertaken the task of compiling this collection of stories.

**Louise P. Sprinkle** loves water and has a surname which is an aptronym. She is in her 70s and works in a number of community roles. She is a mum, a granny, and very fit. She is a secret poet and is amassing a collection of haiku that she has written about her adventurous life.

**Therese Spruhan** is an avid swimmer, writer and photographer from Sydney's Inner West. She chronicles pools, swimmers and places to swim through her blog, *Swimming Pool Stories*, as well as travel articles for *The Weekend Australian* and other writings for anthologies, online and print publications. She also shares pool photos and stories on Instagram @swimmingpoolstories and on Twitter @reseyspru. Her first book, *The Memory Pool: Australian Stories of Summer, Sun and Swimming*, was published by New South Books in November 2019.

**Stephanie Wood** is an award-winning former staff writer at *The Age* and *The Sydney Morning Herald*'s *Good Weekend* magazine. She is now freelancing for publications including *Good Weekend*, *Vogue* magazine and *The Guardian*. She has worked internationally as an editor at London's *The Independent* and *The Asian Wall Street Journal* in Hong Kong. She is a former *Age Good Food Guide* editor and restaurant reviewer. The extracts in this publication are from her compelling 2019 book *Fake*, published by Vintage.

# Acknowledgements

I envy the lone (and sometimes lonely) author whose final task is to thank family and friends and those who assisted in myriad ways with the publication of their book. This book has an additional dimension: to thank the 22 women who wrote, sometimes for the first time, about their experiences at 'The Women's Pool'.

It is important that they be recognized and thanked for their generosity, humour, perseverance and goodwill throughout the two COVID years that have passed since the idea for this book was first conceived. Many have not only written their stories but have given time and other support, from contacting potential writers, editing, proof-reading and chasing photographs, to seemingly endless photocopying of the many evolving versions of the book.

Thanks are also due to the team at Spinifex Press who took on the task of publication, in spite of COVID disruptions, and in a very short time frame. It was important that the book be ready for the summer of 2021–2022 to mark the 100th anniversary of women working together, willingly and joyfully, to accept guardianship of the pool and ensure its continued existence as a safe and special place for women.

Initially a vague suggestion, floated at the pool on a sunny day, the book materialised through word of mouth, commitment to the project and in the fine tradition of the Thursday Married Ladies, over food and wine. Such a pleasure.

*Lynne Spender*
*Sydney*
*September 2021*

*Other books by Spinifex Press*

## Not Dead Yet: Feminism, Passion and Women's Liberation
### Renate Klein and Susan Hawthorne (eds)

What was it like to participate in the Women's Liberation Movement? What made millions of women step forward from the 1960s onwards and join it in different ways? Many of the 56 women in this book were there. They describe how they have contributed in multitudinous ways across politics, the arts, health, education, environmentalism, economics and science and created wonderfully rebellious activism. And how they continue this activism today with determined grittiness. Here are women — all over 70 years of age — still railing against the patriarchal systemic oppression of women, still fighting back. May these riveting tales by the foremothers of the movement inspire young women readers. #NotDeadYet

ISBN 9781925950328

## Making Trouble (Tongued with Fire): An Imagined History of Harriet Elphinstone Dick and Alice C. Moon
### Suzanne Ingleton

In the cold winter of 1875, two rebellious spirits travel from the pale sunlight of England to the raw heat of Australia. Harriet Rowell (age 23) and Alice Moon (age 20) were champion swimmers in a time when women didn't go into the sea; they were athletic and strong in a time when women believed men who told them if they didn't bind their bodies in whalebone corsets they would fall over or ruin their childbearing purpose; and they were in love in a time when many women were in love with each other but held such love secretly, for fear of retribution.

ISBN 9781925581713

## Lillian's Eden
### Cheryl Adam

In *Lillian's Eden*, debut novelist Cheryl Adam takes the reader to Australian rural post-war life through the life of a family struggling to survive. With their farm destroyed by fire, Lillian agrees to the demands of her philandering, violent husband to move to the coastal town of Eden to help look after his Aunt Maggie.

Juggling the demands of caring for her children and two households, and stoically enduring her husband's continued indiscretions, Lillian finds an unlikely ally and friend in the feisty, eccentric Aunt Maggie who lives next door. This rich, raw novel pays homage to friendship and to the rural women whose remarkable resilience enabled them to find happiness in sometimes the most unlikely of places.

ISBN 9781925581676

## Out of Eden
### Cheryl Adam

Pregnant, abandoned and homeless, Maureen battles to survive a Swedish winter until help arrives in the form of a mysterious woman with a veiled past. With the prospect of being deported, Maureen learns who her real friends are, especially when she faces investigations due to her links to a suspected criminal. Meanwhile in Australia, Maureen's family is scrambling to support her when the health of her unscrupulous father declines and he depends on the clever intervention of his estranged family members to salvage both his dignity and finances. An engaging rollicking yet poignant sequel to *Lillian's Eden*.

ISBN 9781925950267

## The Kindness of Birds
### Merlinda Bobis

An oriole sings to a dying father. A bleeding-heart dove saves the day. A crow wakes a woman's resolve. Owls help a boy endure isolation. Cockatoos attend the laying of the dead. Always there are birds in these linked stories that pay homage to kindness and the kinship among women and the planet. From Australia to the Philippines, across cultures and species, kindness inspires resilience amidst loss and grief. Being together ignites resistance against violence. We pull through in the company of others.

ISBN 9781925950304

## Murmurations
### Carol Lefevre

*Shortlisted for the Christina Stead Award
in the NSW Premier's Literary Awards*

Lives merge and diverge; they soar and plunge, or come to rest in impenetrable silence. Erris Cleary's absence haunts the pages of this exquisite novella, a woman who complicates other lives yet confers unexpected blessings. Fly far, be free, urges Erris. Who can know why she smashes mirrors? Who can say why she does not heed her own advice?

Among the sudden shifts and swings something hidden must be uncovered, something dark and rotten, even evil, which has masqueraded as normality. In the end it will be a writer's task to reclaim Erris, to bear witness, to sound in fiction the one true note that will crack the silence.

ISBN 9781925950083

## An Embroidery of Old Maps and New
### Angela Costi

*I can see how I carry Yiayia's war*
*in the ample dunes of my belly,*
*the moment she smelt the guns,*
*she pinched the candle's wick,*
*gathered the startled shadows of her children,*
*flung my baby-mother onto her back*
*and sprinted towards the neutral moon—*

Migration and the memories of women's traditions are woven throughout these poems. Angela Costi brings the world of Cyprus to Australia. Her mother encounters animosity on Melbourne's trams as Angela learns to thread words in ways that echo her grandmother's embroidery. Here are poems that sing their way across the seas and map histories.

ISBN 9781925950243

## I Will Not Bear You Sons
### Usha Akella

*A poem can glisten like a fresh wound.*

Usha Akella pays tribute to the lives of women from cultures across continents, while reflecting on her own life. Her poems are the medium for women who refuse to be silenced. She condenses a calm rage into ferocious words of precision and celebrates the women who have triumphed. All the while a subversive dusting of humour runs through the collection.

This is poetry that cannot be ignored.

ISBN 9781925950281

## The Wear of My Face
### Lizz Murphy

*The Wear of My Face* is an assemblage of passing lives and landscapes, fractured worlds and realities. There is splintered text and image, memory and dream, newscast and conversation. Women wicker first light, old men make things that glow, poets are standing stones, frontlines merge with tourist lines. Lizz Murphy weaves these elements into the strangeness of suburbia, the intensity of waiting rooms, bush stillness, and hopes for a leap of faith as at times she leaves a poem as fragmented as a hectic day or a bombed street.

ISBN 9781925950342

## The Poetics of a Plague: A Haiku Diary
### Sandy Jeffs

*First wave fear is back.*
*Before an end was in sight*
*now there is no end.*

*Trying to make sense*
*of an unravelling world*
*that is downright mad.*

What was it like to live in Melbourne during the 2020–2021 lockdowns? Capturing the day-to-day struggles of lockdown, the daily news, Dan Andrews' 11 a.m. morning press conferences, the tensions between Victorians and the rest of Australia, Trump's chaotic America, the conspiracy theories that circulated and battling her own mental health, Sandy Jeffs takes us through the whirlwind of events in imaginative haiku poems. These became her sanity while the world spiralled into madness.

ISBN 9781925950366

*If you would like to know more about Spinifex Press,
write to us for a free catalogue, visit our website
and subscribe to our monthly newsletter.*

Spinifex Press
PO Box 105
Mission Beach QLD 4852
Australia

www.spinifexpress.com.au
women@spinifexpress.com.au